Fast *Like a* Girl

A Woman's Guide to Using the Healing Power of Fasting
to Burn Fat, Boost Energy, and Balance Hormones

DR. MINDY PELZ
YUNA ADONIS

ISBN: 9798388841773 Paperback

Contents

Foreword

When it comes to the story of my hormones, I don't even know where to begin. I hit puberty at 10 years old and was on the road touring by the time I was 13. Each and every cycle, I experienced severe pain, heavy bleeding, and lots of inflammation. Every part of my body would experience swelling —including my vocal cords—which led to many hospital visits and canceled shows. By my early 20s, I was on a regimen of continuous birth control that was recommended by my gynecologist. Instead of taking the sugar pills in the birth control packet, I would start another pack of pills right away. No period at all meant no inflammation and no canceled shows. Seemed like a good idea at the time.

Then one day, after almost two decades of suppressing my natural cycles, my body decided it wanted to return to its cyclical rhythm. I had undergone a lot of spiritual growth by that point, which enabled me to listen to my gut and ovaries. They told me that it was time to face whatever I had been running from all of these years and allow my body to express what it needed to express. Interestingly enough, my body decided this in December 2019, just three months before we all retreated into our homes because of the pandemic. What I was worried about all those years—losing my livelihood—was about to actually happen, but not in the way I had expected. I'd like to think my body and soul were *that* in tune with what was coming and knew, if I so chose, I could return home to myself . . . pun somewhat intended.

Since allowing my body to return to its natural cycles, the journey back to my instinctive rhythms has felt, at times, like pulling teeth without Novocain, but it has been necessary to discover the fullest expression of my feminine power, the fullest expression of my voice.

You'd think that as a woman who has had music coursing through my veins from the time I was born, rhythm and flow would come easily to me. But to keep up with the patriarchal system of constant production and achievement, I lost touch with the most important rhythm of all . . . my body's innate natural rhythm. I would venture to say that most all of us have, and our bodies, our souls, are whispering, or maybe even screaming, for us to come back home. And for some of us, like me, the homecoming is a little less of a return and more like landing at the center of my truest self for the first time ever.

One day, I was driving down the 101 Freeway in Southern California and listening to a podcast on which I heard Dr. Mindy Pelz on a panel with three other doctors discussing health and wellness within the treacherous times we are currently living. Something about her energy jumped out at me. She was passionate, wise, funny, heart-centered, and seemed genuinely nurturing. Then my inner voice whispered, "You must meet her," but at that moment I didn't know why.

Instead, I scooped up her book *The Menopause Reset*. As a 40-year-old woman headed into, if not already in, perimenopause, I had begun—reluctantly, I might add—to think more and more about the upcoming transition from "Fertile Myrtle" to, well, that part of life everyone tells you is going to be miserable. The part where you bite everyone's head off, have hot flashes, and start to lose your mind. I didn't want my 40s to go down like that, but how could I avoid it when this is what I was taught was almost every woman's experience?

As a "celebrity," I'll admit that there have been a lot of times when the "typical experience" has not applied to my life (especially when trying to get a reservation at a popular restaurant), but there's no way around the humanity of aging and the inevitable shifts that happen in our female bodies.

I have always taken care of my body, but over the last several years I noticed my energy declining. I wrestled brain fog, found myself searching for words when trying to communicate, and forgot why I walked into a room. I also battled severe anxiety and depression over the last decade, which put me on a path of taking medication along with mindfulness and any and every alternative treatment available to me. Still, I felt like I was circling the root of my health issues without any clear solution, and the information I soaked up from Dr. Mindy's book confirmed my suspicions.

I've been very fortunate to work one-on-one with Dr. Mindy, and what she has spent countless hours teaching me is exactly what you are about to learn in the pages that follow. They're lessons that I believe should be taught to women from the time that we hit puberty but aren't. It's time to re-mother ourselves and empower our hearts and minds with the knowledge that allows us to no longer be at the mercy of anything or anyone outside of ourselves when it comes to our health.

If you're wondering what you're getting yourself into by reading this book, that is it: You are about to discover the healing power of your magnificent female form. You are about to learn all the tools necessary to turn on your power for healing, joy, and creation from the most primal, instinctive place—your own body and soul.

Until I met Dr. Mindy, I don't know if I truly believed in the power of my own body to heal itself. But I am a believer now. Whatever challenges you face, know that healing is possible. It doesn't happen overnight. It takes educating yourself—which you are bravely embarking on now—along with love, respect, and dedication for your body's unique needs, but I believe in you and I know, without a doubt, Dr. Mindy does too.

I don't know about you, but as a little girl, the following phrases were said to me repeatedly: "Don't run like a girl," "Don't throw like a girl," and "You hit like a girl." It was as if being a girl or doing anything "like a girl" was "bad" or "wrong."

I wish that little girl knew then that being a girl is a massive superpower! In fact, the woman she's become certainly does now!

This woman knows that her womanhood is sacred; it can wield magic and help her heal herself. It can even help heal the world around her. My prayer is that every woman reading this book comes to know that doing things "like a girl"—especially learning the ways in which to nurture our primal nature—is the path to freedom and the way in which we, as women, begin to help usher in heaven on earth.

—LeAnn Rimes
Grammy-award-winning singer and songwriter
Seeker, speaker of truth, mystic, and overall badass
2022

Introduction

We have never been more in need of a new paradigm for health. In the past few decades, chronic conditions like Alzheimer's, cancer, diabetes, infertility, cardiovascular disease, autoimmunity, mood disorders, and even chronic pain have skyrocketed. What might be the most disheartening about this surge is that many of these diagnoses are happening to women. Yet women are still being given a one-size-fits-all solution that rarely takes into account their hormonal needs, leaving them feeling unheard, out of answers, and, most of all, still sick.

I know this scenario all too well because I was one of these women. At 19 years old, I was overcome by unrelenting fatigue —a fatigue that made it impossible to do even the simplest daily life tasks. At an age when most are thinking about what career to step into, I was struggling to find the energy to even get out of bed. Searching for answers, I found myself sitting in the office of one of the top medical doctors in the world who diagnosed me with chronic fatigue syndrome, a condition for which there was no known cure. He told me it would take years for me to heal from such a debilitating condition and then instructed me to drop out of school, hop onto trial medications, and hope that my body would heal. At that time I was a scholarship athlete with coaches breathing down my neck to get back out on the tennis court; I didn't have time to wait.

We all have moments we look back on and realize that in an instant our life was changed forever. That day I sat in the doctor's office was one of those moments. Like the millions of women who receive dismal prognoses from their doctors, I listened in disbelief. Yet a voice inside me kept telling me there was another way. How could my body be breaking down at 20 years old? If the best chronic fatigue doctor couldn't help me, how was I going to find a way out? That dark moment taught me one important lesson that I have carried forward into my practice today: When your health falls apart, you need just one person to believe in you and give you hope. Luckily for me on that day, that person was my mom. Frustrated with this doctor's advice, she immediately drove me from that doctor's office to a holistic medical doctor. It was 1989, and at that time finding a medical doctor with a more natural approach was almost impossible. His first recommendation? Change my diet. He explained to me how all foods are not created equal: Some foods build up your health and others deplete you. I had been eating the ones that depleted me. He immediately put me on a diet that looked very much like today's wildly popular ketogenic diet.

Within three weeks of adhering to his diet recommendations, I could feel something in my body shift dramatically. Not only was my energy coming back but my brain had more clarity, I started dropping weight effortlessly, and the depressive haze I had been walking around in for months disappeared overnight. I literally felt like someone had given me a miracle cure, yet all I did was change what I was eating.

Why did my body respond so well to these diet changes? What healing power did I ignite with just changing up my food choices? And why did these two doctors have such dramatically different opinions about my path back to health? I was in awe of how quickly my body responded to the new diet changes. It sparked an unquenchable desire to learn what else my body was capable of achieving through the power of food. Yet it also left me wondering how many people are given similar grim prognoses who never get taught the effect food has on our body's ability to heal. This experience ignited a desire in me to help others see the influence something as simple as food can have on their health.

Since then, I have studied and tested almost every popular diet fad that has emerged. You name the new diet trend, I've tested it. I have also spent the past 25 years in the health trenches with thousands of patients helping them discover how important *what* they eat and *when* they eat can be to their health. What all this research taught me is that now more than ever humans are suffering at the hands of poor food choices. Recently the Centers for Disease Control and Prevention published that 60 percent of Americans have one chronic disease, 40 percent have two or more, and 90 percent of the trillions of dollars we spend on health care goes to treating these chronic conditions. Why are we so sick? What has changed in the past 30 years that has us on a collision course with chronic disease? When you look at the root causes of many chronic diseases, you see a common thread—that common thread is poor metabolic health.

Poor metabolic health, often known as metabolic syndrome, is getting a lot of press these days and with good reason. The term *metabolic health* is often used to refer to a person's ability to properly regulate their blood sugar, blood pressure, and cholesterol without the use of medications. Not only does poor metabolic health lead to chronic disease, but it also compromises your immune system. Perhaps the most startling part of having poor metabolic health is that as a culture we have normalized this condition. Many of the hallmark signs that tell us a person's metabolic health is diminishing are often given a label by doctors as "aging," "genetic," or "unavoidable." The signs someone is struggling with their metabolic health are clear: High levels of blood sugar, triglycerides, low-density lipoprotein (LDL) cholesterol, blood pressure, or an increasing waist circumference are all telling you that your metabolism is struggling. A classic sign of a failing metabolism that is rarely addressed is a person's inability to go without food. This is referred to as hypoglycemia, but your brilliant body has a reserve energy system that should activate in the absence of food to give you energy, mental clarity, and tide you over until you can get to your next meal. If you are struggling to go more than four hours without food, it is time for a metabolic tune-up.

In 2018, a study emerged from the University of North Carolina at Chapel Hill declaring that only 12 percent of Americans are metabolically healthy. And it's not just Americans: More than 800 million people worldwide currently live with obesity. According to the *British Medical Journal*, in many countries obesity is now killing more people than smoking.[1] What might be most disturbing is that the fastest-growing sector of the population living with obesity is children. Childhood obesity is predicted to increase by 60 percent in the coming decade, reaching 250 million by 2030. The medical costs associated with this rise in obesity are expected to exceed $1 *trillion* by 2025. Respected medical journals like *The Lancet* are even declaring that due to the strong correlation of metabolic disease to worse COVID-19 outcomes, metabolic health needs to be our number one focus globally in the post-pandemic era.[2] Yet our current efforts to prevent and treat metabolic challenges like obesity are glaringly inadequate. Our approach to this growing problem needs to change. Poor metabolic health is not just a number on the scale or an elevated lab finding; it is a person in crisis. Each health crisis doesn't just affect that individual; it impacts that person's family, our communities, and, as the pandemic has taught us, the world at large. We are all in this metabolic mess together.

As dismal as our current metabolic situation may be, there is a clear path out. It's a path that doesn't take time and won't cost any money. It's backed by science and can be done by anyone, anywhere, anytime. That tool is fasting. Although the art of fasting is not a new health concept, in recent years people have discovered that fasting is the quickest path back to better health. In my quest to help patients improve their health through nutrition, I stumbled upon multiple studies proving the efficacy of fasting. I became so enamored with what the science was saying about how our bodies heal in a fasted state that I incorporated it into every one of my patients' treatment plans. The results were astounding. I had never seen the body heal so quickly just by tweaking something as simple as when a person eats. This left me wondering, *If fasting was so powerful for my patients, could this be a tool that everyone could use?*

Throughout my 25 years in practice, I have consistently seen that two of the biggest hurdles people come up against when trying to get well are time and money. Fasting takes care of both. I became so obsessed with this reemerging ancient health tool and the results I was witnessing that I decided to teach the science of fasting on my YouTube channel. I quickly discovered that many people, especially women, were also thirsty to learn how to fast effectively. Three years and 900 videos later, I have been on the front lines witnessing a burgeoning health trend that has patients and doctors alike clamoring to learn more. In the years since I have been teaching fasting, hundreds of thousands of healing stories have been shared on my channel. What has been clear is that people are falling in love with the results they experience when they fast.

As you will soon discover, the studies on fasting are impressive as well. Respected scientific journals such as *The New England Journal of Medicine*, *Cell Metabolism*, *Nature*, and *The British Medical Journal* consistently publish new evidence proving why fasting works so well. These papers show how fasting helps with every aspect of metabolic health, from weight loss and high blood pressure to insulin resistance, inflammation, and lowering cholesterol. We also have scientific evidence that fasting repairs our gut microbiome, improves neurodegenerative diseases like dementia and Alzheimer's, reboots a struggling immune system, and can power up happiness neurotransmitters like dopamine, serotonin, and GABA.

While the scientific evidence is clear that fasting heals, there still exists one huge blind spot: A one-size-fits-all approach to fasting doesn't work, especially for women. As exciting as it is that more people are incorporating intermittent fasting into their lifestyle, three critical questions have emerged that are not being addressed.

The first is, How long should someone fast? Intermittent fasting is typically thought of as going 13 to 15 hours without food. Yet many follow the research that's been done on 16:8 fasting—16 hours of fasting alternating with 8 hours of eating. Meanwhile, one of the most famous fasting studies revealed that a three-day fast can kill precancerous cells and reboot your whole immune system. As these scientific articles become more mainstream, and fasting becomes more popular, a lot of opinions are being tossed around on how long a person should fast. This makes it incredibly confusing for many to determine how long they should fast, if they should fast every day, and whether they are even fasting correctly. As you learn to thrive in a fasted state, it's tempting to go longer. But is longer better? Often there are no clear answers.

The second question is, What foods are best paired with fasting? Many have fallen so in love with fasting, they forget that food heals too. Yet it's the rhythm of moving in and out of feasting and fasting that creates the greatest metabolic change. Fasting experts have been focusing primarily on the healing that happens within the fasting window, leaving fasters in the dark as to the healing importance of food when they do eat. This is a challenge since many people are still eating a Western standard diet that is packed with chemicals, sugar, and inflammatory fats. As contradictory as this may sound, food should not be left out of the fasting conversation. When you pair the right foods with fasting, miracles happen—especially for women.

This brings me to the third and most important question that needs answering: Do women need to fast differently than men? This is a pivotal question because women are highly influenced by the monthly and menopausal swings of hormones. The intricacies of our sex hormones—estrogen, progesterone, and testosterone—require that we pay closer attention to spikes in cortisol and insulin that can happen with an increase in stress, exercise, food, and, yes, even fasting. When we use fasting to flip our metabolic switch, we need to do it in sync with our hormones. Although men are hormonally driven as well, their hormones are not as sensitive to these spikes. For a woman to realize the full health benefits of fasting, she needs to know *when* and *how* to flip her metabolic switch in accordance with her hormonal cycles.

Yet like in many aspects of health care, women are often left out of the conversation. Multiple fasting books are teaching a one-size-fits-all approach to fasting, leaving women with more questions than answers. Podcasts, social media posts, and blogs discuss the need for women to fast differently, but very few are teaching women *how* to fast differently. This presents a huge challenge. If a woman decides to jump into a fasting lifestyle and doesn't time that fast to her menstrual cycle, adverse symptoms may appear such as hair loss, rashes, anxiety, missed menstrual cycles, thyroid problems, and trouble sleeping. These are all symptoms that can be avoided when a woman learns how to fast for her unique body. Done properly, fasting can resolve so many conditions women are struggling with. The same goes for menopausal women who may no longer have a cycle but still have hormonal needs. We need to address what their fasting lifestyle should look like. The list of women looking for fasting answers to their hormonal conditions is long. Women with polycystic ovary syndrome (PCOS), women using IUDs with very little evidence of a menstrual cycle, and the hundreds of thousands of women who are struggling with infertility—these are all women who need to adjust a fast to their specific needs. And they need resources to guide them.

In an effort to help, I started teaching the intricacies of fasting and how to time a fasting lifestyle to hormonal needs on my YouTube channel. I mapped out six different fasting styles (ranging in length from 13 to 72 hours) and two different food programs (what I call ketobiotic foods and hormone feasting foods) that can be timed to women's menstrual cycles. I also created a tool called the Fasting Cycle that lets a woman choose the right fasting length and food style to correlate with her menstrual cycle. And for women both with and without a cycle, like menopausal women or women on birth control with minimal flow, I created a step-by-step 30-Day Fasting Reset that varies their fasting lengths and food choices to balance their hormones while improving their metabolic fitness. If there is anything that these women have taught me, it's that once a woman knows how to build a fasting lifestyle around her cycle, she becomes unstoppable.

It's these women who have inspired me to write this book. On these pages, you will find the proven strategies, condition-specific protocols, hacks that make fasting easier, and tools that I have used to help hundreds of thousands of women just like you thrive with a fasting lifestyle. I have split the book into three parts, starting with the science behind fasting and metabolic switching. Knowing the *why* behind fasting is key for your success. In Part I, I also guide you through a brief lesson on how your hormones work. This is the lesson you should have been given at age 13, and I am excited to give it to you now. Marrying the science of fasting to the magic of your hormones is pivotal for your fasting success. In Part II, I dive into food principles that will never let you go metabolically astray again. Nutrition can be complicated; I want to simplify it for you. In this part, I also introduce you to the two eating styles— ketobiotic and hormone feasting—that you will match to your fasts. You will also learn how to use the Fasting Cycle to sync your different-length fasts to your menstrual cycle. Finally, in Part III, you will learn how to customize fasting to your life, including using a 30-Day Fasting Reset, specific protocols you can use if you are trying to overcome a condition, and hacks that will make fasting easier. One of my favorite concepts to teach—how to break a fast—is outlined in this section as well. No matter where you might be in your fasting journey, I know you will find resources here that will help you move the needle with your health.

Just like my mom was that beacon of hope for me years ago, I want this book to be your guiding light as you learn to use fasting and take back control of your health. This book will teach you exactly how to do that. Women have been underserved by the medical community for too long, and I am excited to share with you the promise fasting provides for each one of *us*.

PART I

THE
SCIENCE

CHAPTER 1

It's Not Your Fault

Your body is a nearly perfect machine. It's made up of more than 30 trillion cells that act like a unified team, working hard to make sure you thrive. Each individual cell is like a little factory that produces energy by burning fat, metabolizing glucose, and manufacturing antioxidants. These cells know when to power you up with energy so you can perform a task, and when to slow you down so that you can rest. When you eat, they gobble up the nutrients you have provided for them and use those nutrients to do the tasks needed to keep you functioning at your best. If food is not available, they switch over to an alternate fuel source to ensure you have the strength and mental clarity to continue functioning. When the receptors on the outside of these cells sense hormones circulating in your blood, they open up their gates and let these hormones in. They efficiently adapt to any physical, chemical, or emotional influences that you throw their way. Pretty spectacular, right?

Here's the challenge: They need your support. They need certain nutrients to function properly—nutrients like good fats, amino acids, vitamins, and minerals. When they don't get that support, they stop being able to do their job. This is why trendy diets have failed you. Most quick-fix diets work against your cellular design, making it impossible to get a longer-term, lasting result and setting you up for numerous health problems that accelerate aging and put you on a path to chronic disease. In this chapter I want to walk you through five ways in which diets have led you down a twisty path—one that you can course-correct at any time. I call these "the failed five": They include calorie restriction, poor food quality, constant cortisol surges, increasing toxic loads, and one-size-fits-all approaches. Once you understand these five diet failures, you'll see that you have been on one heck of a health roller-coaster ride. Most diets have blindly disconnected you from your body's design, leading you straight into the arms of frustration, self-doubt, and distrust with your body. This dieting madness needs to stop. The results you want can happen when you step away from the constraints of this diet culture, understand how your amazing body was designed, and embrace a new health paradigm that works with this incredible female body you get to live in.

Before I jump into specifics, I want you to honor yourself for a moment. I know that you've watched friends succeed at popular diets and tried to mimic their results only to discover you couldn't achieve the same success. I know how frustrating it is when you go to your doctor's office searching for answers to a health crisis only to be shamed and told you need to lower your BMI. I get how exhausted you are with one-size-fits-all pill solutions that don't work. I realize that the hours you have spent at the gym trying to exercise yourself to better health with little result have left you wondering whether there is something wrong with you. You can let go of all of that now. Those beliefs won't serve you on this new health journey you are about to embark upon.

As you let go of guilt and shame, also know that you are not alone. Too many women are feeling the way you do. According to the CDC, 41 percent of women 21 and older are obese. Forty-five percent have high blood pressure. One out of two will develop cancer in their lifetimes. One out of five will develop Alzheimer's. One out of nine will get type 2 diabetes. One out of eight will develop a thyroid problem. Eighty percent of all autoimmune conditions occur in women.[1] As a collective group, we are struggling. These are our sisters, mothers, grandmothers, aunts, friends, co-workers, bosses, and community leaders. We are the caretakers of our families and our communities. At a time when the world needs us to be at our best, we are grappling with poor health, feeling unheard by doctors, and are searching for answers to reclaim our power. Healing begins when you can forgive yourself for the past. As you read through these five failures, know that there is a good chance it's not your fault that past diets haven't worked for you. Let go of any feelings of failure, scary diagnoses that you've been labeled with, or limiting beliefs you may have accumulated along your path. Letting go of such negative thoughts will serve you as you step into this new healthier version of yourself.

THE FAILED FIVE

#1 Calorie-Restriction Diets

If there is one myth I could permanently extract from your mind, it's that counting calories keeps you thin. You have been taught that eating less and exercising more will give you lasting health and happiness. We call this approach to dieting the "calorie in, calorie out" theory, and it's one of the hardest ways to lose weight permanently.

Why? Every time you eat less and exercise more, you change your metabolic set point. Your set point is where your body maintains its weight within a preferred range of calories. Old-school thinking said your genetics determined this set point. The lucky ones got a higher set point, while the unlucky were stuck with a lower set point. New evidence is proving this to be wrong. It turns out that you train your set point, and when you eat less and exercise more you lower your set point threshold. This is where low-calorie diets failed you. Because each time you lowered your threshold, you made it more difficult on yourself to eat any other way. When you go back to eating more calories or working out less, the pounds come back on much easier because you are above your set point threshold. Maddening, right?!

Unfortunately, this has been women's go-to diet for years. Often this approach does produce a temporary result, seducing you to keep coming back for more. Yet, tragically, over time your body will fight the reduction in calories by increasing hunger signals to your brain and slowing down your metabolism. Because of the change it makes to your set point, it's incredibly hard to succeed at low-calorie diets long term. Unwinding your beliefs around calorie restriction can be hard. If this is you, let's look at one of the most famous studies on calorie restriction ever done: the Minnesota Starvation Experiment. Although it dates back to the 1960s, this experiment is still revered as the most prominent study ever done on the physical, emotional, and social changes that happen when the human body is put into a calorie-restricted state for long periods. Over a 13-month period, 36 men were given progressively lower amounts of food until they settled in on a 1,500-calorie diet. When administering this low-calorie diet, researchers noticed several dramatic changes to the physical and mental health of their subjects. First, they became preoccupied with the thought of food to the point that they couldn't stay focused on daily tasks. They also became depressed, anxious, listless, and hypochondriacal, and began to withdraw socially. Sound like your experience with your last diet? As concerning as this sounds, perhaps the most startling result was what happened when food was reintroduced to the study participants. When the experiment was over, the participants continued to experience mental health problems. They also quickly gained back the weight they had lost—and packed on an extra 10 percent of their body weight. Poor mental health and extra weight is not a dieter's dream, yet so many of us have unknowingly replicated this study. On so many levels, this study proves the damage calorie restriction does to our health.

#2 Poor Food-Quality Choices

Forty years ago, the American government declared a war on fat. Concerned that fat was contributing to cardiovascular disease, they advised people to stay clear of all kinds of fats, especially saturated fats and cholesterol. This declaration catalyzed the low-fat movement, forcing the food industry to develop "fat-free" foods. With the removal of fat, however, the food industry had a big obstacle to overcome—taste. Fat makes food taste great. So the food industry replaced fat with sugar and flavor-enhancing chemicals in its products, which caused obesity rates to skyrocket. In the 1960s, fewer than 14 percent of Americans were considered overweight; today that number is closer to 40 percent, with projections forecasting that 50 percent of Americans will be obese by 2030.

When you see a low-fat label on a product, quickly put it back on the shelf. Equate low fat to high-sugar, highly toxic ingredients—two things that will quickly cause you to pack on the pounds. Why did these new trendy low-fat food products cause us to gain weight? The irony is that we are now discovering that ultra-processed foods, like those found in many popular diets, make us insulin resistant.

Insulin resistance is a term that is getting a lot of press these days, largely because so many people are struggling with obesity and diabetes. But what is it exactly? Insulin resistance is a condition in which your cells can no longer successfully use insulin as a hormone to escort the sugar from your food into your cells. When your cells become unable to use glucose for fuel, not only will you experience a depletion in energy but they will store the unused glucose as fat. This is the root cause of metabolic syndrome, which is defined as having three out of five of the following components: obesity, high blood pressure, high blood triglycerides, high blood sugar, or low levels of HDL cholesterol. When reports emerge showing that only 12 percent of Americans are metabolically fit, we know we have a collective health problem.

Let's take a look at how insulin is supposed to work. Insulin is your sugar-storing hormone. Your pancreas releases this hormone after you eat a meal to escort the sugar from that meal into your cells. The more sugar-dense a meal, the greater the insulin release. A constant influx of insulin will flood your cells, overwhelming the receptor sites that allow the hormone to perform its job. Receptor sites are the gates on the outside of our cells that open up to let hormones in. The more insulin that floods these gates, the more congested these gates become—like a big cellular traffic jam. It is at this moment that your cells become deaf to insulin. Much like you may constantly ask your spouse to do a household chore—the more you ask, the less they seem to hear you. Your cells do the same thing with insulin. Once they stop responding to insulin, both the excess insulin and sugar will be stored as fat. Diets that don't help you manage this insulin response will set you up for failure.

#3 Spiking Cortisol Surges

Cortisol is the enemy of insulin. You can't be in a state of stress and build health at the same time. When cortisol goes up, so does insulin. How does this work? Let's go back to the calorie-restriction diets you may have tried in the past. The rigidity of these diets often creates stress, spiking your cortisol levels. You start reducing the number of calories you eat, which makes you hungry and irritable. This new agitated state creates a fight-or-flight reaction in your brain, and your brain responds by releasing cortisol into your bloodstream, telling your body there is a crisis at hand. Your body responds to this crisis signal by shutting down digestion, halting fat burning, and raising your glucose levels so that you are physically prepared to handle this stressful situation. As your glucose levels go up, insulin rises to meet the new sugar demands. Once more, a surge of insulin overwhelms your cells. The crazy part is that all of this happens without a single nibble of food entering your mouth.

Repetitive cortisol spikes will impede your dieting results. Any rigid diet that you have to consistently muscle your way through will keep cortisol high for potentially too long. But cortisol spikes don't just happen because your boss overloads you with work, or you have an argument with your spouse. Often cortisol spikes can happen when you hop on a diet that is restrictive and hard to fit into your lifestyle. Cortisol can also rise when you are overexercising, trying to force your body into a state of health. I have even seen women who get so obsessed with their results with fasting that they go longer and longer in a fasted state, creating a constant flow of cortisol. Cortisol is the elephant in the room that is often not addressed on popular diets. You can't be in constant states of stress and improve your health at the same time.

And you don't need to be on a diet to have cortisol mess you up. Day-to-day stresses can give you cortisol spikes. We call it a *rushing woman's lifestyle*, a term coined by Dr. Libby Weaver in her book *Rushing Woman's Syndrome*. That's because a woman's body is much more sensitive to swings in stress than a man's body. We are hormonally designed to procreate, and when stress goes up it signals a massive hormonal shutdown to occur. When a stress response gets triggered, our brain thinks a tiger is chasing us. It will reorganize all our hormones in that moment so that we are neurochemically prepared to run from the tiger. This new configuration of hormones often means that our sex hormones drop and insulin rises. Once this occurs, it doesn't matter how great your diet is, how many hours you spend at the gym, or what detox program you are on, your health will suffer.

Many of the diets you've been on don't address the need to keep cortisol in check. You may have noticed this when implementing a new diet while living your rushing woman's lifestyle.

#4 Exposure to Toxic Ingredients

Toxins make you fat. Seriously, they do. So much so that a new category of fat-inducing chemicals has been given its own name—obesogens. When your body gets an influx of these chemicals it doesn't know how to break them down, so it stores them as fat. Remember that the next time you look in the mirror and villainize the stubborn weight that won't go away; rethink the purpose of that fat. It's not there to stress you out. Your body literally didn't know how to break down the chemicals in your food, so it placed it in your fat stores so that it wouldn't harm the organs that keep you alive. It's a brilliant system your body has created for your long-term survival.

What chemicals are considered obesogens? The list is long, but these are the five worst: BPA plastics, phthalates, atrazine, organotins, and perfluorooctanoic acid (PFOA). Although the chemicals on this list are abundant in our foods, water, beauty products, cleaning products, cookware, and even our clothing, for the sake of this book I will be talking mostly about food-sourced obesogens. Common obesogens found in food include monosodium glutamate and soy protein isolates. Both are commonly found in weight-loss shakes. Much like a flood of insulin blocks receptor sites on the outside of your cells, so do obesogens. They, too, block the hormonal receptor sites, making it impossible for your hormones to enter your cells to do their job. This can dramatically blunt everything from thyroid hormones to insulin from entering your cells, leading to more weight gain, fatigue, and erratic mental health.

Detoxing these chemicals out of your body can be the answer to a variety of health challenges, including weight-loss resistance, thyroid problems, and autoimmune conditions. When you stop to read the ingredients of many prepackaged diet foods, you'll see that they are laden with chemicals. Don't be fooled by the marketing of these foods. Fancy words like *all natural*, *low calorie*, or even *keto friendly* can be grossly misleading; foods labeled as such might be filled with obesogens. In Chapter 6, I will share the list of ingredients to avoid, so that you can do so effortlessly.

#5 One-Size-Fits-All Approaches

There is no one perfect diet for everyone, and in this book I'll show how that is particularly true for women. We all have different hormonal needs at different times of our lives, and our diet needs to accommodate that ebb and flow. One of the biggest harms that has ever been done to women's health is the perpetual belief that we *all* should be on the same diet. You will learn in Chapter 6 that each one of your sex hormones has different food requirements. Estrogen, for example, loves a low-carbohydrate diet, while progesterone wants you to keep your carbohydrate load a little higher. This means you need to vary the foods you eat to match the ebbs and flows of your hormones. But how many diets have done this for you? If you are a cycling woman, most diets have you eating the same way all month long, possibly working against the needs of your hormones. If you are a postmenopausal woman with low hormonal production, diets are not geared toward giving you food solutions that maximize your age-appropriate hormone production. The diets you have most likely been on have been structured with a one-size-fits-all approach.

The exciting part of accepting this is you will see that as a woman there is a better way to approach our relationship with food, one that is built on adapting our diet to our menstrual cycles. This is a skill that we should have been taught when we first started puberty and should be modified for us as we go through menopause. The massive amount of hormonal issues women face today—like infertility, breast cancer, and polycystic ovary syndrome—can often be alleviated by learning to tune our lifestyle needs to our monthly cycle.

As you begin to step into this new paradigm, I want to point out one other place this one-size-fits-all approach destroys us. It's in comparison, notably, comparison with each other. Instead of trying to create our own beautiful unique health path, we watch other women and the results they get with their diets and assume our body can achieve the same result. All too often we determine our self-worth by comparing ourselves to another woman's highlight reel. This is as damaging to our bodies as any of the five failed diet strategies listed above. As you learn to fast like a girl, keep in mind that even though we are all living in a female body, we don't all have the same lifestyle needs. When a friend hops on a diet, gets great results, and we try to mimic those results, we set ourselves up for failure. Every woman is on her own unique hormonal journey. Finding a diet that is customized to our hormones is pivotal if we want to succeed at our health. Thus far, the rules of the dieting game have not been in your cellular favor. As you move through the pages of this book, I encourage you to keep exploring the idea that there is a path back to health that is unique to you. If you ever doubt the power that lives within your own body, come back to this foundational truth: Your body is always working for you, not against you. I realize it might not feel like that right now, but as you learn to sync up your lifestyle choices with your hormones, you will discover how effortless building health can be. If symptoms show up or you struggle to overcome a health obstacle, ask yourself, "What is my body trying to say to me?" It's easy to keep searching outside ourselves, blaming our poor health on genetics, doctors, diets, or wrong medications. But this outward blame hasn't made us healthier. As women, if we are going to take our health back, we need to turn within.

The magic of fasting starts with an inward journey. As you move into the next chapter, which details the science behind fasting, I want you to keep in mind your body was designed to self-heal. You are about to learn that you have come preprogrammed with a menagerie of healing responses, like autophagy, that your body will tap into when you fast. Combine your fasting and food choices to your hormones and you will discover a level of health you may have never known to be possible.

This is exactly the path that one of my YouTube subscribers, Sarah, took. Doctors told her she was on a fast path to diabetes and that she should lose weight by cutting calories and choosing low-fat, sugar-free foods. She tried this strategy for years only to find herself packing on more weight with each diet attempt. Frustrated with empty answers from her doctor about her poor metabolic health, she turned to YouTube to solve her own health challenges. (That alone should tell you something about the level of frustration many women are experiencing.) Deep in searching metabolic solutions for herself, she stumbled upon my fasting videos. Most of the fasting information she had seen was from male experts who had said that fasting wasn't good for women. Sarah was so excited by the principles I was teaching on YouTube that she binge-watched my videos over and over again. She was tired of feeling powerless and wanted to get these fasting concepts down. After enough research, Sarah jumped in. She began the process of fasting like a girl, building a fasting lifestyle that was unique to her. Within a year's time she had lost 80 pounds and was off five of her medications. (Her doctor was so in awe with her results that he wanted to learn more about what she had done. Sarah sent him to my channel, where he dove into the research and started encouraging his female patients to fast, recommending my videos as a resource to learn how to fast properly. Pretty soon the rest of the women in his practice started getting similar results to Sarah.)

You are powerful beyond your wildest imagination. Starting now, you can step into a new possibility. This journey will require you to make three perspective changes. These are changes you can make immediately. The first is to let go of the past. Any unsuccessful tries you've experienced with dieting are behind you. Forgive yourself. The second is to promise yourself you will never fall victim to the five diet failures again. They no longer serve you. And the third is to place your heart around this new vision of health you are about to create for yourself. Get ready for a whole new paradigm of health that will serve you in so many beautiful ways. I am beyond excited to guide you through this process. Let's get started.

CHAPTER 2

The Healing Power of Fasting

For hundreds of thousands of years, our hunter-gatherer ancestors spent their lives having to search for food. Long before farming or agrarian cultures existed, humans were forced to fast involuntarily. Then once they found food they feasted, followed by more days of fasting. Cycling between times of famine and feasting was the way of life for our prehistoric ancestors. Because of this, many scientists believe that these harsh evolutionary conditions created a new genotype within humans—a genotype that gives our bodies the necessary cellular tools to adapt to the cycles of fasting then feasting. Called the "thrifty gene" hypothesis, it speculates that this genetic coding still exists in us today.[1] It posits that when we don't mirror our ancestors' feast-famine cycling behaviors, our health suffers. Supporters of the thrifty gene hypothesis believe that this is a pivotal reason why obesity and diabetes rates have skyrocketed. Our current approach of eating all day, without ever dipping into periods of fasting, has us going against our own genetic code.

A look back in history reveals several examples of how the human body thrives in a fasted state. Although done for spiritual reasons, Ramadan fasting is one of the greatest examples of how the human body positively adapts to long windows of time without food. In fact, some of the best fasting research has been birthed out of studying the Muslim community during Ramadan. We also have evidence that in the 5th century B.C., Hippocrates, the father of modern medicine, used fasting as one of his primary healing tools. During a time when humans believed disease was punishment by the gods, Hippocrates boldly declared that diseases were caused naturally, believing that environmental factors, diet, and other living habits were to blame. Hippocrates used healing therapies that were built around strengthening the body's own innate resistance to disease, and one of those therapies looked much like intermittent fasting and the ketogenic diet. "People should exercise on an empty stomach, their meat should be fat as the smallest quantity of this is filling, and they should only have one meal a day." He saw it as the answer to everything from epilepsy to strengthening resistance against the plague.[2]

How does this work? Is fasting built into our genetic code? Was Hippocrates on to something thousands of years ago? In this complex modern world, where food is available 24/7, is fasting the key healing tool we've forgotten? Current science is proving that answer to be yes. In this chapter I want to explain what a fasted state looks like in this modern day, the healing mechanisms that are getting turned on while in this state, and how the science is revealing that longer fasts can turn on more healing switches within our cells that may have a multitude of benefits to us as women.

The best place to start is to understand what it means to fast, and to understand that you have two fuel systems that your cells get their energy from so you can function: sugar and fat. The first system, called the sugar-burner energy system, gets activated when you eat. Eating food raises your blood sugar. Your cells sense this influx of sugar in your blood and use that sugar, called glucose, as fuel for the thousands of functions they perform. When you stop eating, your blood sugar drops. This slow decline of glucose in your blood triggers your cells to switch over to the second energy system—called the ketogenic energy system, or what we lovingly call the fat-burner system. Very much like a hybrid car that switches from gas to electric for fuel, this switchover is when the fasting benefits begin. Although everyone will make this switch differently, research shows that it takes about eight hours after your last meal for your body to shift to its fat-burning system.

If you have never gone longer than eight hours without food, there is a likelihood that you may have never experienced the healing benefits of your fat-burner energy system. One of the most comprehensive analyses ever done on the science of fasting was published in *The New England Journal of Medicine* in December 2019.[3] The authors reviewed more than 85 studies and declared that intermittent fasting should be used as the first line of treatment for obesity, diabetes, cardiovascular disease, neurodegenerative brain conditions, and cancer. It also stated that intermittent fasting has anti-aging effects and can help with pre- and post-surgery healing. This meta-analysis highlighted several key cellular healing responses that happen when we periodically flip our metabolic switch and move into our fat-burning system. These cellular healing benefits include:

- Increased ketones
- Increased mitochondrial stress resistance
- Increased antioxidant defenses
- Increased autophagy
- Increased DNA repair
- Decreased glycogen
- Decreased insulin
- Decreased mTOR
- Decreased protein synthesis

Numerous studies are also proving that outside of the above cellular changes, the most important part of improving your metabolic health is changing *when* you eat, not *what* you eat. The first such study in *The Journal of Nutrition, Health & Aging* in 2018 showed that obese individuals saw dramatic metabolic improvement despite eating whatever they wanted as long as they ate that food within an 8-hour eating window, leaving 16 hours for fasting.[4] *Cell Metabolism* published findings in 2020 revealing that the same diet eaten in a 10-hour period had a greater metabolic effect on a person than if they spread that diet out over a 14-hour time period.[5] Both studies show very clearly that when you condense your eating window, leaving more time for fasting, you will:

- Reduce total body fat percentage
- Reduce visceral fat
- Reduce waist circumference
- Lower blood pressure
- Decrease LDL cholesterol
- Decrease hemoglobin A1c

In a modern world where we have been conditioned to eat low-quality food all day long, research like this gives me hope that we can begin to undo much of the metabolic damage that is causing so many to struggle with poor health. Changing the time period in which we eat is more important than the actual quality of the food we eat. This is great news if we are to improve our metabolic health. Everyone can learn to take this fasting step. It doesn't take time or financial resources to fast. And you don't have to change your diet to better your metabolic outcomes. Something as simple as compressing your eating period will yield incredible results! These studies prove the benefits that allowed our prehistoric ancestors to thrive when food was absent. Can you see why so many have become smitten with fasting? Not only are you burning energy from fat, accelerating weight loss, lowering blood pressure, cholesterol, and insulin, but the more often you access this fat-burning state, the more repair can happen in your body. It's much like sleep. When you are getting consistent sleep, your body has a chance to heal at a deeper level than when you are awake. A great night's sleep is one of the most powerful healing tools you can access. The same goes for fasting. Each time you put your body into a fasted state, you are giving your body the opportunity to heal. Fasting is not like any other diet. It is not a moment of deprivation; it's a gift you give yourself that will allow your body and brain to recover from the stressors of the modern world.

To better understand how this works, I want to highlight some of the major healing responses your body triggers while you are fasting so that you can get to know them better.

Increases ketones

Ketones are an organic compound the liver makes when your blood sugar drops. Ketones are an alternative fuel source for your cells when glucose is not readily available. A hallmark sign that your body is burning energy from fat is the presence of ketones. There are many healing benefits to having low levels of ketones surging through your system. Ketones are reparative, meaning they will go to certain tissues in your body and regenerate them. Specifically, they repair nervous tissue. This is incredibly helpful with any neurodegeneration that may have occurred in the brain. Ketones have the power to regenerate damaged neurons that carry information throughout your brain, improving your memory and ability to retain new information, as well as giving you increased focus and mental clarity.

Ketones are also a preferred fuel source for your mitochondria —the parts of your cells that make your energy. In Chapter 3, I will dive more into the power of your mitochondria, but in regard to ketones, if your mitochondria are sluggish and not providing the necessary energy to function at your best, ketones will power them back up. It's the ultimate mitochondrial reset. This energy is much different from the energy you feel when you eat. When operating from the sugar-burner system, you will often feel your energy go up and down. Ketone energy is much different; it is consistent, giving you both physical and mental clarity throughout your day.

The wonders of ketones don't just stop with brain repair and energy. Ketones will also go up to the hypothalamus of your brain and turn off your hunger hormone. This is a large reason why the more you fast, the less hungry you will become. As your brain senses ketones when you click into your fasted state, it will use those ketones to kill your hunger. Many fasters use this decline in hunger to extend their fasts a little longer, getting even more of a healing benefit. The rise in ketones also triggers the release of a calming neurotransmitter called GABA. This neurotransmitter has an anti-anxiety effect on your brain, leaving you feeling more relaxed despite not eating any food.

For many, ketones are what they are chasing with their fasting lifestyle. You feel limitless when your body makes ketones. If you fear how you feel when you fast, remember that once your cells have made the switch over to this fat-burning state and ketones are on the scene, your energy and mental clarity will increase. It's the opposite of any diet you have ever been on. When you train your body to make ketones, fasting will not only get easier but more healing will occur with time.

Increases autophagy

If there is one cellular process that has drawn so many to fasting, it's autophagy. When your cells register dipping blood sugar while in a fasted state, this incredible repair process kicks in. Why do your cells do this? To make themselves more resilient. Without the influx of glucose coming in, your cells respond by making themselves stronger. Autophagy improves cellular resilience in three ways: detox, repair, and the removal of diseased cells.

The concept of autophagy was brought to the world's attention when Dr. Yoshinori Ohsumi, a Japanese scientist, won the 2016 Nobel Prize in Physiology or Medicine for his landmark research, which revealed that in the absence of food our cells get stronger, not weaker. Instead of looking for nutrients outside the cell when food is scarce, that cell turns within and eats what's inside. When you break down the word *autophagy*, it means "self-eating." Oshumi's work was so profound that it sparked thousands of other studies to follow, helping us understand why autophagy is such a necessary healing state for the human body.

Because of its ability to clean your cells up, autophagy was first associated with the fasting world as being analogous with detox. Although autophagy is a form of detox, it only detoxes organic materials within the cells. Over time our cells accumulate a variety of damaged organelles, proteins, oxidized particles, and harmful pathogens. This accumulation causes our cells to become dysfunctional. When in a state of autophagy, our brilliant cells will detox these malfunctioning parts out of the cell, thus revitalizing them. This cellular reboot is a large reason why so many fasters feel younger and more vibrant the more times they dip into an autophagy state. Food will typically pull you out of autophagy, while longer fasts put you back into this healing state.

One of my favorite recent studies done on autophagy was published in 2020. It looked at the possible benefits of autophagy as a tool for priming the immune system to fight the coronavirus that sparked the COVID-19 pandemic. Viruses don't have an energy system, so when they enter your body, they must work off your energy system. If your cells are in a sugar-burner state, viruses will enter your cells, fuel themselves on sugar, and gain energy that allows them to multiply quickly. If a virus enters a cell that is in a state of autophagy where it doesn't have sugar to consume, it will lose energy and its ability to replicate. The sneaky part of a virus like COVID-19 is that once it enters your cells, it shuts down autophagy so that it can replicate faster. Fasting can help restore autophagy's ability to shut down viral replication.

The other form of detox that autophagy will perform for you is getting rid of old, worn-out cellular parts. Remember how your cells are like little factories with lots of moving parts working to your advantage? Well, these parts can get overworked and worn down. Once that happens, they can't do their job effectively. Ineffective proteins and organelles within your cells accelerate the aging process, suppress your immune system, and can tank your energy. When you fast and stimulate autophagy, you trigger your cells to remove these lagging parts.

As beautiful as this system is, there is one thing that autophagy doesn't detox: synthetic, man-made chemicals like plastics, phthalates, or perfluoroalkyl and polyfluoroalkyl (PFAS) and other "forever chemicals" (so called because they do not break down naturally, staying in the environment forever). The process of autophagy also can't recycle out naturally occurring heavy metals like lead or mercury, which can do damage to your brain and hormonal system, not to mention destroy your mitochondria.

When your cells are in a state of autophagy but sense a malfunctioning cell, they will initiate cellular death, a process known as *apoptosis*. Cells packed with toxins often go rogue, turning into cancer cells. Destroying this cellular situation is key for your long-term health. Dipping into states of autophagy on a regular basis is a helpful tool not only for building high-performing cells but also for removing damaged cells that lead to disease.

The last key feature of autophagy is its ability to repair your mitochondria. Known as mitophagy, this is a healing response triggered by fasting in which your cells will eliminate dysfunctional or damaged mitochondria, counteracting degeneration and inflammation that can lead to an array of common health challenges including cognitive disabilities, muscle weakness, chronic fatigue, and impairments in hearing, vision, and liver and gastrointestinal function.[6]

Bottom line: When you fast, you put your cells into both a state of autophagy and ketosis, creating an amplified healing state that will have your body performing better than you may have ever dreamed possible. This is the magic of fasting!

Decreases glycogen and insulin stores

If you've been eating a high-sugar diet for years, your body has had to store all of that extra sugar somewhere. It stores it in a form of sugar called glycogen. There are three key places your body puts this excess sugar: muscles, liver, and fat. Think of it like when you make a big shop at the grocery store and not all of the food you bought will fit in your refrigerator, so you store it in a freezer in your garage. This is what your body will do with excess glucose. It stores it as glycogen in your fat. Once you run out of food in the kitchen, you reach for the extra food in the garage. That is what your body does when fasting. You force it to go find the excess sugar it's been storing for years and use that for fuel. The glycogen stores in your muscles are easy to get to through exercise, specifically high-intensity interval training and strength training. But how do you get to the liver and fat stores? This is where fasting really shines as it is one of the most effective ways to release glycogen stores in your liver and fat.

And you will want to get that excess glycogen out of your liver. Your liver is one of the hardest-working organs in your body; it's burning fat, breaking down hormones, and making lots of good cholesterol to fuel your brain. Once inundated with sugar, your liver becomes inefficient at these pivotal jobs, which can lead to diabetes, fatty liver disease, and high cholesterol. Fasting is a fabulous way to get the liver to release excess glycogen so that it can function at its best.

In addition to ridding yourself of glycogen in your liver, by fasting you'll get rid of all the sugar that got stored in those fat cells and was left there for future use. Fasting gives your cells a reason to use that sugar. This is why so many fasters get lasting weight-loss results—they are finally able to undo all the damage done from previous diets.

And there's more. Excess glucose is not the only thing your cells release when you fast. Fasting also forces your body to release excess insulin. As mentioned in the previous chapter, insulin spikes every time you eat. If you eat a high-sugar, high-carbohydrate meal, you will experience a large insulin spike. Do this several times a day for years and you end up flooding your cells with insulin, thus making them insulin resistant. Like it does with extra glucose, your body has to store this excess insulin somewhere, so it packs it away in your liver and fat. Once again, the more you put yourself into a fasted state, the more you force your body to go find those insulin stores and metabolize them for excretion.

What does all of this mean for you? It's simple: Change when you eat and you will undo the years of damage that poor living has done to your health. We've spent all these years debating which diet is best for humans, and it turns out, according to the science, that the best outcomes to our metabolic health happen not when we change what we eat but by the simple act of compressing our food intake into a smaller eating period of 8 to 10 hours. Think about this for a moment. Every diet you have ever been on has started with changing the foods you were eating or limiting the amount of calories you consumed, often putting you on a weight-loss roller coaster and perhaps even leading to great irritability and depression like the Minnesota Starvation Experiment proved. Fasting changes the dieting game. That result you have been searching for through dieting can now be achieved through fasting.

Increases growth hormone production

Our body's growth hormone is our fountain of youth. When we are younger we have this hormone flowing through us in spades, but as we age its production dries up. Growth hormone production peaks at puberty, then makes a slow decline until it completely stops at 30. Ask anyone who is over 30 and they will tell you that this was the moment when the aging process started to kick in.

Growth hormone performs three key functions. The first is that it helps you burn fat, especially around the midsection. The second fabulous process that growth hormone provides is muscle growth. Have you noticed that your muscle-building efforts in the gym yielded results more quickly when you were younger? I can't tell you how many women over 40 I have heard complain about the muscle loss that occurs with aging. Once again, the disappearance of growth hormone will accelerate the muscle loss you experience with age. Lastly, growth hormone supports healthy brain growth. When you were younger your brain needed it to help it learn new life skills. After 30 you have learned most of the skills necessary to perform daily life tasks, so this hormone isn't needed anymore.

But what if you want to burn more fat, increase your muscle size, and have the brain power to learn a new skill? Once again, fasting comes to the rescue. Depending on the length of your fast, decreasing blood sugar levels stimulates your body to make growth hormone fivefold, giving you back that youthful feeling.

Resets dopamine pathways

Every time you eat something yummy, you are getting a dopamine hit. In fact, sometimes you get the dopamine rush just *thinking* about that food. When we eat all day long, we get dopamine hits left and right. This raises what we call your dopamine baseline. As this baseline gets raised, you need more dopamine-producing experiences to feel good. Just like you can become insulin resistant from too much insulin flooding your cells, you can become dopamine resistant from using food all day long to feel good. In fact, the research on dopamine and obesity shows that some obese individuals keep eating all day not because they are hungry but because they need more food to get a normal dopamine response. Obese individuals not only need more dopamine to feel the satisfaction of food, but as they age they have less dopamine receptor sites available to receive the dopamine.

Food isn't the only source of dopamine. We can get it from visual or audio triggers. The noise your phone makes telling you that you have a text message gives you dopamine. The followers and likes on your social media give you dopamine hits. Even the DoorDash guy ringing your doorbell minutes after you ordered food from your couch provides a dopamine rush. In today's world, we are dopamine saturated.

The good news is that several studies show you can reset your dopamine pathways with different-length fasts. Not only does fasting stop the age-related decline of dopamine receptors that obese individuals experience, but several types of fasts can actually make your dopamine receptors more sensitive. In some cases new dopamine receptor sites are formed, increasing your overall feelings of contentment.

Repairs the immune system

One of the most famous fasting researchers, Dr. Valter Longo, brought the three-day water fast to the world's attention. His notable study was done on patients going through chemotherapy; he wanted to see if fasting would help repair the decimated white blood cells that occur with a chemo treatment. On the third day of a water fast he saw something miraculous happen: Old, worn-down white blood cells died off and a new, energized group formed. It was a reboot to the immune system that anyone going through chemotherapy needs. That happened because of the release of stem cells into the bloodstream at 72 hours of water fasting. Remember, the body gets stronger the more it fasts. It does this to energize your body so it can go find food. The stem cells that are released at 72 hours ensure your body is working at its best so that your chance of finding food is at its best. Specifically, the job of stem cells released at 72 hours is to identify the worn-down white blood cells and make new ones to replace them.

Improves your microbiome

At the center of most fasting discussions is the incredible changes that happen to us on a cellular level. But did you know your body houses 10 times more bacteria than it does human cells? And these microbes have a tremendous influence on how your human cells function. It is estimated that you have more than 4,000 different microbial species living in and on you, 90 percent of which live in your gut. They help pull vitamins and minerals out of your foods, make neurotransmitters like serotonin to keep you happy, break down estrogen so it's ready for excretion, and constantly scan your cells for inflammation that might need to be lowered. Trillions of bacteria are all hard at work supporting your cells so they can function at their best.

One emerging challenge humans are now faced with is that our modern lives are destroying our beneficial microbes. Everything from the foods we eat, the medications we take, and the stress we encounter to even the Wi-Fi that infiltrates our homes is destroying these helpful bacteria. It is a well-known fact now that one round of antibiotics will destroy 90 percent[7] of your gut bacteria—90 percent! How many rounds of antibiotics have most people been on, 10 . . . 20? I have had consultations with patients who tell me that they have been on more rounds of antibiotics than they can count. We also have evidence that the simple act of taking one round of antibiotics can change your delicate microbial balance to favor storing your food as fat.

Two of the most abundant bacteria phyla you have in your gut are Bacteroidetes and Firmicutes. Research is proving that obese individuals have more Firmicutes than Bacteroidetes, causing them to store more of their calories as fat.[8] You can give two people the same diet and the one whose ratio of Firmicutes to Bacteroidetes is out of balance will gain weight, while the other person won't gain a pound. Obesity has also been linked with decreased gut microbial diversity compared to lean individuals.[9]

Weight loss, neurotransmitter production, breaking down estrogen—these are only a handful of jobs these microbes perform for you on a daily basis. Microbes have a hand in everything from how hungry you get to the foods you crave. The more microbial diversity you have, the lower your appetite will be.[10]

Depressed yet? Well, here's the good news: Fasting brings back the health of these microbes. It does this in four ways: It improves microbial diversity, moves microbes away from the gut lining, improves the production of bacteria that change white fat into brown fat, and regenerates stem cells that will repair the gut lining. (Brown fat is the fat that keeps you warm. It is also an easier fat to burn for energy.) All four of these factors are key if you are looking to lose weight.

According to Dr. Emeran Mayer in his book *The Gut-Immune Connection*, when microbes move farther away from the gut lining, better glucose regulation is achieved. This is called microbial geography, and fasting can help create an environment in which the microbes are equally distributed, allowing them to perform at their best. Fasting can also impact the microbes that help turn white fat into brown fat. White fat is that stubborn fat that is hard to burn. Typically, it is subcutaneous fat and the most visible to see, so it's the fat that you most likely want to get rid of first. The best way to lose this fat is to convert it into brown fat. Brown fat has more mitochondria within each cell and therefore produces more heat, making it easier to burn.[11] When you fast, you increase the microbes that can make this conversion.[12] Amazing, right?!

Lastly, there is impressive scientific evidence out of the Massachusetts Institute of Technology proving that fasting can regenerate intestinal stem cells.[13] Stem cells are cells that can go to any injured body part and repair it. With regular 24-hour fasts, you reinvigorate the stem cells that live in the lining of your intestinal tract, allowing them to repair any damage that may have happened from a poor diet, stressful living, or numerous rounds of antibiotics.

We also have evidence that longer fasts, like a five-day water fast, can dramatically impact your gut bacteria, specifically the bacteria that influences blood pressure. A study published in *Nature* revealed that when participants went on a five-day water fast, it precipitated a microbiome change that contributed to a reduction in their blood pressure. The interesting part of this study was that the test subjects were split into two groups: one that fasted before the diet change and one that didn't. Both groups followed the DASH diet, well known for lowering blood pressure, but one group preceded the diet change with a five-day water fast. This group saw the greatest change in blood pressure, which suggests that fasting could be a superior lifestyle modification over food changes to alleviate high blood pressure.

Reduces the reoccurrence of cancer

In 2016, *The Journal of the American Medical Association* released an observational study that looked at more than 2,000 women between the ages of 27 and 70 who had undergone conventional breast cancer treatment. After analyzing this large group of women for four years, researchers determined that when women fasted 13 hours or more, they had a 64 percent less chance of recurrence of breast cancer. This is largely because fasting created a significant decrease in hemoglobin

A1c, an indicator of blood glucose levels, and C-reactive protein, an indicator of inflammation. Very few drugs can offer that kind of result. This is how miraculous the body can be when fasting.

Years ago, I helped a patient named Lani who was diagnosed with metastatic breast cancer at age 40. Given three months to live, this beautiful woman did everything she knew to do to extend her life. Her philosophy for discovering how to heal herself was to leave no stone unturned. Because of her tenacious spirit and quest for learning ways to help herself, she turned a three-month prognosis into 11 years of vibrant life. One of my biggest takeaways from Lani's journey was that it is far easier to prevent a disease than to reverse it. When I read studies like the one above, it reminds me that we don't have to have a cancer diagnosis to benefit from the findings that this study offers us. A daily commitment to longer fasting not only helps women who have had breast cancer not get a recurrence but may also help women avoid getting a breast cancer diagnosis in the first place. New fasting studies are emerging daily, and studies like this one give us hope that we will see more scientific evidence that fasting is a go-to tool in the fight against many cancers.

Have I got you excited now? I sure hope so! Are you starting to gain a deeper understanding of why so many women are enthusiastic about the miracles they see with their health as they fast? With this better understanding of all the general benefits of fasting, let's dive into the specific benefits of different-length fasts so that you can choose the best fast for you.

SIX DIFFERENT-LENGTH FASTS

Not all fasts are created equal. With that in mind let's break down six fasts, the research behind them, and when to use them for your own healing journey. The six different fasts are:

- Intermittent fasting: 12–16 hours
- Autophagy fasting: starts at 17 hours
- Gut-reset fast: 24 hours
- Fat-burner fast: 36 hours
- Dopamine-reset fast: 48 hours
- Immune-reset fast: more than 72 hours

Intermittent Fasting (12–16 hours)

This is the most popular style of fasting. Most people's definition of intermittent fasting is going anywhere from 12 to 16 hours without food. The easiest way to understand how this works is to walk through what a 24-hour period might look like when incorporating intermittent fasting into your life.

Let's say you finish dinner at 7 P.M. You don't eat or drink anything after that point so that your blood sugar starts to decline. If you delay your breakfast the next day until 10 A.M., that's 15 hours of fasting. A general rule is that your liver will switch on and start making ketones somewhere around eight hours from the last morsel of food or sip of drink you put in your mouth. Somewhere between the 12- and 15-hour mark, as your body is making energy by burning fat, ketones flood your bloodstream. The first place those ketones go to is your brain, turning off hunger and giving you a boost of physical and mental energy. Your cells begin to move into a state of autophagy, repairing, detoxing, and regenerating themselves. As your liver continues to sense the absence of glucose, it keeps releasing glycogen and insulin stores by breaking down more fat. Dip into these fasted states repeatedly and you will start to see long-term improvement in metabolic markers like blood pressure, fasting glucose and insulin, hemoglobin A1c, and C-reactive protein. The bacteria in your gut will also shift as bad bacteria dies off and good bacteria regrows. This improvement in your microbial makeup will lower blood pressure, allow your body to make more mood-enhancing neurotransmitters, and help your blood sugar balance more efficiently.

Think of intermittent fasting as your entry point into fasting. It is the easiest fast to fit into your life and will yield you the quickest results. Many people turn to intermittent fasting when they feel weight-loss resistant or they get fed up with yo-yo dieting. When done properly, intermittent fasting is a huge step forward in getting your body to go back to burning energy from fat instead of sugar.

If you are new to fasting, here's your first goal: Eat your food in an 8- to 10-hour time period, leaving 14 to 16 hours for fasting. Start by pushing your breakfast back an hour. Do this for a week, then push your breakfast back for another hour, and keep extending your fasting window until you are comfortably fasting for 14 hours. Some people find that for weight loss it's better to move their dinner up an hour instead of moving breakfast back. That works too; it's personal preference. Eating too late and then going straight to bed can impede weight loss. Either way, the goal is to train your body to adapt to a longer period without food, with your first major fasting ledge to grab on to being 14 hours.

Although intermittent fasting benefits just about everyone, there are some very clear reasons to use intermittent fasting specifically:

- If you want to lose weight;
- You're experiencing brain fog;
- You're suffering from loss of energy.

Weight loss

There's no doubt that intermittent fasting will unstick your weight. Not only does the science continually prove this, but I have had a front-row seat to hundreds of thousands of people who have lost weight just by fasting 15 hours a day. This happens because you are flipping that metabolic switch and for the first time getting your body to make energy by burning fat. Once your body is using that fat-burning energy system, weight tends to drop off quickly.

Brain fog

For most people, their fat-burning energy system will start to make ketones around the 15-hour mark of intermittent fasting. Ketones will supercharge the brain, gifting you with great mental clarity. It often feels like someone turned on a light switch in your brain; you will feel focused and clear. Even though the longer fasts will only enhance that mental experience, intermittent fasting is where most people start to see the release of the brain fog they may have been dealing with for too many years. Because of the power of ketones on your brain, intermittent fasting is an amazing tool to use before a big test, speech, or any performance where you need mental clarity.

Loss of energy

Of your two energy systems, the fat-burning one will provide you with the greatest energy boost. The energy you get from eating is often dependent upon the quality of the meal you put together. High-carbohydrate meals might give you an immediate burst of energy but then can cause your energy to crash soon after. Protein-rich meals might not elevate your energy as quickly but can often be a great way to lift your energy gradually without experiencing the crash. Each meal you eat will provide you with a different energetic experience.

This is not the case with the fat-burning energy system. When you are intermittent fasting and switch over to making energy from fat, you will feel a certain zing to your energy. Many fasters can tell you the moment in their day when they feel this switch happen. It's like you've had a cup of coffee without any of the negative jitters that may accompany it. Your energy with ketones is consistent, clear, and often feels never-ending.

I promise you that once you train your body to intermittent fast, it will feel effortless. Most women find this length of fast easy to incorporate, even into the busiest of lifestyles.

Autophagy Fasting (17–72 hours)

There is much debate about at what hour of fasting autophagy kicks in.[14] I like to think of autophagy as a dimmer switch that slowly gets turned on around 17 hours and reaches its brightest peak at 72 hours. The healing benefits of autophagy are vast, but the simplest way to know when it's time to extend your fast to trigger autophagy is when you want to:

- Detox;
- Improve brain function and cognition;
- Prevent a cold;
- Balance sex hormones.

Detox

Just finished a vacation during which you overindulged? This is the perfect time to throw in a few days of autophagy fasting. It's a great tool to use when your cells have been inflamed and worn down from a few days of bingeing. Think of autophagy as this magical eraser that will undo the damage a poor diet created within your cells. After the holidays or post vacation is the perfect time to lean in to this cellular healing tool. Autophagy can repair the mitochondrial damage that occurs when there is an influx of toxins flooding your bloodstream.

Improve brain function and cognition

The brain benefits of intermittent fasting build with autophagy fasting. The neurons in your brain are highly influenced by autophagy, making it a powerful tool for slowing down neurodegenerative aging, improving memory recall, enhancing mental cognition, and experiencing greater mental clarity and focus. Lean in to autophagy fasting when your mind is unfocused, memory is sluggish, or you need more mental power to learn a new skill.

Prevent a cold

Autophagy fasting has amazing powers over the immune system. Remember this when you go into a panic after someone has sneezed on you. Empower yourself in that moment by fasting longer so that you can stimulate autophagy. When your cells are in a state of autophagy, viruses and bacteria that enter them can't replicate. This is key during cold and flu season, a pandemic, or anytime someone around you is sick. Any fast that's longer than 17 hours will trigger autophagy and help you stay immune strong.

Balance sex hormones

Your ovaries are very responsive to autophagy. This makes autophagy fasting useful during your perimenopause years, when you are trying to get pregnant, or with a diagnosis of polycystic ovary syndrome (or PCOS) as it can bring health back to your ovaries and balance out your hormones.

Studies done on PCOS are proving that a key root cause of this hormonal condition is dysfunctional autophagy. In 2021, a small study of 15 women with PCOS revealed that five weeks of restricting their eating window to an eight-hour time frame not only improved menstruation but also contributed to weight loss, a reduction in inflammation, and lower insulin levels—all hallmark challenges of PCOS. Because the thecal cells surrounding our ovaries are so influenced by autophagy, hormone production is best balanced using a longer fast.

My clinical experience has taught me that going into states of autophagy is incredibly helpful for declining hormones that are often experienced with perimenopause and infertility. Cycling in a longer autophagy fast once or twice a week often helps maximize sex hormone production.

Gut-Reset Fast (24+ hours)

If I had a favorite fast, the gut reset would be it. Here's why: It's easy, time efficient, and has a major impact on your microbiome. When you are in a fasted state for 24 hours or more, it's long enough to get a burst of stem cells released into your gut to repair its inner mucosal lining, which may have been damaged from years of chronic inflammation.[15] This is the magic length of fasting to start seeing significant changes in your gut health. This fast is the first point at which your body will make stem cells, and those stem cells will find worn-out cells and bring them back to life. People pay large amounts of money to get stem cells injected into their joints, skin, and injured body parts in hopes of regenerating those areas. You can get a similar effect by fasting.

Ninety percent of your microbes live in your gut. Extending your fast to 24 hours invigorates these microbes that are critical to your immune system and will help make neurotransmitters that keep your brain happy, calm, and focused. Clinically the three most common times I use this longer 24-hour gut-reset fast are to:

- Counteract antibiotic use;
- Offset birth control use;
- Help tackle small intestinal bacterial overgrowth (SIBO).

Counteract antibiotic use

As I mentioned above, antibiotics kill 90 percent of the bacteria in your gut. These are both good and bad bacteria. Although the bad bacteria that caused the infection is gone, the good bacteria that supports your health is decimated as well.

Integrating a couple of 24-hour fasts recharges those stem cells so they can repair the terrain of your intestinal tract, which antibiotics may have altered. This gives you a microbial do-over. Combine a 24-hour fast with foods that feed your gut good bacteria and you can undo the damage that years of antibiotic use has done to your body.

Offset birth control use

The birth control pill kills microbial diversity, contributes to a leaky gut, and creates an environment where yeast grows. A leaky gut is a condition in the gut where the tight junctions of the thin mucosal lining open up and toxins, undigested food, and harmful pathogens can enter the bloodstream, causing the body to have a systemic inflammatory response. Many women have been on the pill for decades and are left with the nasty side effects of a leaky gut as a result. Just because you stop using this medication doesn't mean the gut damage it has done goes away. This is where 24-hour fasting can really save you. The more opportunities you have to go into this length of fast, the more you'll repair the damage that the pill may have caused. For a damaged gut, the healing that can happen with 24 hours of fasting is more powerful than any antibiotic, fancy supplement, or fancy diet.

Help tackle SIBO

Small intestinal bacterial overgrowth, known as SIBO, is one of the most difficult gut conditions to overcome. Unlike the large intestine, the small intestine usually doesn't have any bacteria, so when bacteria does start to grow there, problems arise. A hallmark sign of SIBO is bloating when you eat fibrous foods like vegetables. There are very few supplements or medications that create a lasting effect in treating this condition, but 24-hour fasts shine in this moment because they let your own body do the healing. You aren't feeding those bacteria anything that would cause them to grow more; you are just changing the environment within the gut, which allows your microbes to come back to homeostasis, the state of optimal functioning for the human body.

Fat-Burner Fast (36+ hours)

No doubt fasting has taken the world by storm because of what an effective weight-loss tool it has been for so many. As exciting as the weight-loss benefits of fasting can be, there is a subset of people who fast every day, often eating only one meal, and the scale still won't budge. In an effort to help, I started leading some women whose bodies seemed resistant to weight loss through 36-hour fasts. It worked like magic! That length of time turned on a fat-burning switch they weren't able to get with shorter fasts. You will want to lean in to a 36-hour fast every once in a while to:

- Minimize weight-loss resistance;
- Release stored sugar;
- Reduce cholesterol.

Minimize weight-loss resistance

Many women will tell you that they are weight-loss resistant. For most of these women, this resistance will be resolved with a shorter intermittent fast. The fat-burner fast is really geared for the woman who has tried the shorter fasts with little to no weight-loss result.

Why does this length of fast work so well for weight loss? Remember all those years you ate poorly? Well, your body had to store that extra sugar somewhere, so it stored it in both your liver and fat. In order to trigger the release of that stored sugar, you may have to stay in a fasted state longer than 24 hours, and clinical experience has shown me that 36 hours is the magic number.

A *Cell Metabolism* study published in 2019 looked at the power of a 36-hour fast followed by a 12-hour eating window, a style of fasting often referred to as alternate-day fasting (ADF). This particular study was the largest of its kind. When subjects followed an alternate-day fasting regime for 30 days, it was noted that ketone production continued, even when they ate in 12-hour windows. They also saw a reduction in cholesterol and inflammation with the ADF group.[16] The most exciting part of this study was the fat loss that happened around the midsection in the ADF group.

I realize if you are new to fasting that it can be hard to wrap your mind around not eating for 36 hours. But as you become more comfortable with fasting, and because of studies like this and the results I witnessed in my community, there may come a time that you feel ready to stay in a fasted state for 36 hours to invoke a deeper metabolic healing response.

Release stored sugar

Often when women fast they notice that their blood sugar goes up. This is the body's way of releasing sugar that it previously stored in tissues, specifically the liver, fat, and muscle tissue. Many women won't see lasting weight-loss results until that stored excess sugar is released. There are a handful of ways of going after that stored sugar. The first is to keep fasting. It's that simple. The more you fast, the more opportunities you give your body to find and release the sugar it has stored in your tissues for years. If you want to speed up the process and get that stored sugar to release more quickly, throw some 36-hour fasts into your fasting mix. This length of fast is magic for applying just the right amount of stress on your body so that it has no choice but to let that sugar go.

Reduce cholesterol

Cholesterol is made in your liver. When your liver has been dealing with high influxes of sugar, inflammatory fats, and toxins, you will often see your cholesterol levels rise. The liver also makes ketones. Longer fasts, like a 36-hour fast, can not only jump-start the liver's ability to make ketones but also repair the liver so that it stops overproducing cholesterol. Often when a woman goes onto a low-carbohydrate, high-fat diet, she will see her cholesterol rise. This indicates that her liver is congested and needs some fasting help. Research plus clinical experience has proven time and time again that when you go into a 36-hour fast, you force the liver to clean up its act and make ketones for fuel. As the liver is healing during this longer fast, you will see cholesterol levels come down. Doing this length of fast once a month can often be the cholesterol solution you've been looking for.

Dopamine-Reset Fast (48+ hours)

This length of fast is what I consider a mental health boost. As mentioned previously, fasting can repair dopamine receptor sites, create new dopamine receptors, and improve your dopamine pathways.[17] There is also scientific evidence that fasting longer than 24 hours makes your dopamine receptors more sensitive.

For the past several years I have been leading my online community through different-length fasts. I call it Fast Training Week, where as a community we practice fasting for different lengths of time. And every time, the 48-hour dopamine fast seems to improve people's mental health more than any other fast. The interesting part of this length of fast is that the fast itself doesn't bring mental clarity immediately; rather it's in the weeks that follow when your whole dopamine system is regenerated that you will feel the benefits. Often just one 48-hour fast will do this for you. When do you want to lean in to a 48-hour fast? When you want to:

- Reboot dopamine levels;

- Lower anxiety levels.

Reboot dopamine levels

Not feeling joy in your life is often not a circumstantial situation but a neurochemical one. As I mentioned previously, sometimes we have been so flooded with dopamine-rich events throughout our day that our dopamine baselines get elevated, making it harder to experience those joyful moments. Dopamine is your molecule of more. Although a dopamine high can be exhilarating, a rush of this neurotransmitter never leaves you feeling satisfied. This is when a good old-fashioned dopamine-reset fast can reboot your dopamine levels and bring back your joy. It doesn't take a lot of 48-hour fasts to reset this system; often one a year can do the trick.

Lower anxiety levels

When you are in a state of anxiety, you are operating from a part of your brain known as the amygdala. The amygdala's job is to keep you safe, so when you operate from this part of your brain you tend to think of all the things that are wrong in your life. This puts you in fight-or-flight mode, often causing you to react to every stressor you experience. There are two ways to move your brain out of this place; one is by stimulating your prefrontal cortex and the other is by making the neurotransmitter GABA. A 48-hour fast helps your brain accomplish both of these tasks. Most people notice that at the 48-hour mark their brains are calmer and not squawking at them as much.

Immune-Reset Fast (72+ hours)

This fast is often referred to as the three-to-five-day water fast. The reason many go up to five days is because at 72 hours in a fasted state your body regenerates stem cells.[18] Revitalized stem cells are able to find injured body parts and make them anew again. After three days of fasting, new and improved stem cells can have a dramatic healing effect on aging cells. And you will keep making those stem cells until you eat again. Many people like to keep going with their fast, extending it to five-plus days to maximize stem cell production. I encourage people to lean in to this length of fast when they want to accomplish one or all of these four things:

- Ease a chronic condition;
- Prevent chronic disease;
- Alleviate pain and stiffness of relentless musculoskeletal injuries;
- Slow down the effects of aging.

Ease a chronic condition

I realize that a three-day water fast is not for everyone, but it can be a miracle for anyone dealing with a major illness. Because the research on three-day water fasts was originally done on patients going through chemotherapy, it's been proven that patients with a cancer diagnosis can really use this type of fast to give an overhaul to their immune systems. On the third day of a water fast, old, ineffective white blood cells will be destroyed and new ones will emerge stronger and more resilient. This can be miraculous for anyone going through an experience of cancer, unrelenting autoimmune conditions like rheumatoid arthritis, stubborn musculoskeletal injuries like a frozen shoulder, and lifestyle-induced type 2 diabetes.

Prevent chronic disease

Although not well researched, many experts believe that three-day water fasts done one to two times a year will help you get rid of any cancer cells that may be building up in your body. We all have cancer cells within us. What stops those cancer cells from turning into tumors is a properly functioning immune system. Physical, emotional, and chemical stressors wear down our immune system, rendering it ineffective in detecting these cancer cells. Because of the efficacy of a three-day water fast on rebooting your immune system, many like to use this length of fast as a preventative tool.

Alleviate relentless musculoskeletal injuries

Stem cells that are revitalized as a result of three days of water fasting aren't there just to repair your immune system. Stem cells can repair any injured body part, making this a great length fast for combating chronic musculoskeletal injuries such as arthritis. In my clinic, I have seen this length of fast work like a charm for the most stubborn injuries. In recent years, stem cell injections have become a trend among aging athletes who are trying to overcome the chronic degeneration that can occur to joints from repetitive exercise. These stem cells can cost up to tens of thousands of dollars per injection. With my patients who suffer with these relentless injuries, I like to have them try a three-day water fast first to see if their body can make their own stem cells and heal the injured body part.

I even tested it on myself with an Achilles tendon injury I had that wouldn't go away. I tried everything to heal it—rest, massage, chiropractic treatments, herbs, acupuncture. You name it, I tried it. Yet it still persisted. As a last resort I went on a five-day water fast, and it healed. No joke, the pain was gone and never has returned. That's the power of a longer fast.

Anti-aging

Stem cells turn back the hands of time. Because they can repair all different types of cells in your body, when you get a surge of them your body finds the tissues that have the most degeneration and heals those first. The beautiful part of the stem cell surge that results from a longer fast is that your body will determine which tissues are most in need of repair. It takes at least 72 hours for stem cell production to begin. A lot of fasters who want anti-aging effects go a few days past the 72-hour mark, giving their body as much of a stem cell surge as possible for healing, knowing that once they eat, the stem cell production turns off.

Hopefully you are seeing the bigger picture of how powerful fasting can be for your health. I will continually remind you that the goal of fasting is to find your unique groove with it. The science is compelling, but matching it to your health goals, lifestyle demands, and hormonal needs is key. In order to do this effectively, I want to take you on a journey of understanding at a deeper level metabolic switching, your hormonal profile, and what it looks like to vary your fasting lengths. Metabolic switching is such an important concept to your health that I have dedicated a whole chapter to it. It is a fasting concept that is often overlooked, but once you truly understand it you will not only level up your health but find a rhythm with your fasting lifestyle that will serve your personal health goals best.

CHAPTER 3

Metabolic Switching: The Missing Key to Weight Loss

One of the amazing things about your body is that it is constantly regenerating itself. In fact, every seven years you get a whole new body. Old cells will die and new cells will form, each body part replicating at a different pace. For example, your skin cells replace themselves every two to four weeks. The cells that line your stomach replace themselves every five days, while it takes your liver cells anywhere from 150 to 500 days to completely replace themselves.

Here's the catch: Sick cells will replicate more sick cells. Once a cell becomes diseased, it will keep replicating that diseased cell. You have a lot to do with how your body responds to your day-today activities. Your physical, emotional, and chemical stressors will determine whether these cells stay in a healthy, vibrant state or move into a more diseased, fatigued state. This shift in cellular health can accelerate aging, contribute to your growing list of symptoms, and deplete your life of joy. But you can reverse it.

If you want to move out of these diseased states, you need to start making healthy cells again. The most effective way to do this is to use fasting as a tool for metabolic switching—your cellular fountain of youth.

Metabolic switching is a shift from utilizing glucose for energy to fatty acid–derived ketones for energy. The act of going in and out of two fuel sources elicits a healing response. We currently have many popular examples of metabolic switching: ice plunges, hypoxic breathing rituals, and fasting. In all of these scenarios you are pushing your body to an edge where your cells are forced to repair. As extreme as this sounds, your body was primally designed for metabolic switching.

If we examine the daily lives of our hunter-gatherer ancestors, we find evidence that they thrived despite going through times when food was sparse. Why have our bodies been able to thrive through harsh food conditions? Let's look at a classic scenario our ancestors went through. When they woke up in the morning, it's not like they had a fridge full of food, so they had to go hunt for their sustenance. They needed fuel to search and hunt. But remember, they hadn't eaten since the day before, so their bodies had entered a fasted state in which they made ketones that provided them with the necessary resources to function and the clarity and focus to find the food they needed to survive. These ketones energized and repaired the inner workings of their cells so they would be successful at finding food. When they found food, they gathered around the fire and feasted, most likely on meat and plants, stimulating a cellular growth process called mTOR that allowed their brains and muscles to strengthen. The next day this feast-famine cycle started all over again. Week after week, month after month, our ancestors exemplified how metabolic switching increased their chances of survival.

In today's modern world, we are not given many opportunities to metabolically switch. We have access to food 24/7. From the moment we wake up to the moment we go to bed, we have food available to us. We don't even have to leave the couch to have food appear. We binge-watch our favorite Netflix series, decide we are hungry, grab our cell phone, and use an app like DoorDash to order food. Within an hour that food appears at our front door. Although these modern conveniences feel luxurious at the moment, they are making us metabolically sick. It's time to mimic our primal ancestors.

Let's take a closer look at all the specific areas in which metabolic switching benefits you. Daily metabolic switching repairs your body. For example, your liver loves when you metabolically switch because when you go into periods of fasting, you force the cells of the liver to release stored sugar, allowing it to heal and repair.

Follow up that fast with foods that support liver health, like bitter vegetables such as dandelion greens or radicchio, and you now put this vital organ into both healing and metabolic healing states.

The gut also benefits when you metabolically switch. When you go into longer fasting states, such as 24 hours plus, you repair the mucosal lining of your gut, making it a better environment for good microbes to grow—microbes that will help you metabolize food and hormones. If your gut were a garden, fasting would be the tool you would use to till the soil and pull the weeds so that the ground would become fertile enough to grow beautiful flowers. Prebiotic and probiotic foods are the flowers you want to plant in your garden. You need both the tilling and the planting in order for the garden to flourish.

Your brain also thrives when you move in and out of your two metabolic states. Your neurons—the trillions of messengers of the million bits of information that move throughout your brain every second—get damaged from toxins and excess sugar. When you fast you begin to repair these neurons, allowing information to get carried proficiently from one neuron to the next. These neurons also have nutritional requirements: A diet rich in vitamins, minerals, proteins, and fatty acids will supply them with the fuel they need to keep you focused and mentally clear. Fasting cleans up these neurons, while nourishing food builds them strong again. Both metabolic states are needed in order for the trillions of neurons in your brain to perform at their best.

Why does metabolic switching work so well in repairing and healing your body? There are four major healing effects that it taps into:

- Alternating between autophagy and mTOR
- Creating a hormetic stress
- Healing your mitochondria
- Regenerating neurons in your brain

Alternates between autophagy and cellular growth

When you metabolically switch, you alternate between two cellular healing processes—autophagy and mTOR. These two processes are like night and day. You can't be in both states at the same time. We discussed autophagy in the previous chapter. On the opposite side of autophagy lives a cellular process called mTOR. This is your cellular growth pathway. When you stimulate this, you can grow cells that contribute to hormone production, build skeletal muscles, and even regrow insulin-producing beta cells in the pancreas. There is a dark side to mTOR, though. If you are constantly stimulating mTOR by eating all day, you are putting your cells into a state of growth too often. Every cell in your body has a life span. The more you stimulate growth, the shorter that cell's life span will be. Too much mTOR stimulation ages your cells quickly, while a little bit of mTOR stimulation is beneficial.

One hotly debated concept of fasting is that it can break down muscle. This is where metabolic switching really shines. When you fast too much, constantly stimulating autophagy, you can cause too much breakdown of skeletal muscle by using the glucose stored in your muscles for fuel while in a fasted state. Once you eat again, glucose will be added back to your muscles, giving them the necessary fuel to grow strong again.

When you eat all day, not leaving enough time to be in a fasted state, you constantly put your cells in a state of growth, accelerating aging. But moving in and out of fasting and fed states will allow you to get the benefit of both of these healing pathways. Fasting part of the day will clean up your cells and following that up with good healthy food will provide the necessary nutrients to help your cells grow strong. Many women discover that metabolically switching helps them lose weight and build muscle at the same time. Time that switch to your menstrual cycle and you are now not only losing weight but also building muscle and supporting good hormonal production as well.

Creates a hormetic stress

The second reason metabolic switching works is because it creates a hormetic stress on your body. A hormetic stress is a low-dose stressor that encourages your body to adapt, forcing your cells to become healthier and more efficient.

You may have experienced a hormetic stress during a workout. When you first do a new workout it's stressful to your body. Take weightlifting, for example. With each new increase in weight, you break down your muscle, forcing it to build itself stronger. If you stay at that same level of weight, it will no longer be stressful to your body and the strength improvement stops. Most personal trainers know this and will keep varying a workout to push the body to new levels of adaptation. Hormetic stress happens with fasting, as well. When you first go from six meals a day to intermittent fasting you stress your body by forcing it into a healing state. In my 30-Day Fasting Reset I will show you exactly how to take that first hormetic step into your fasting lifestyle. Often when women first go from eating all day to eating only two meals a day, they notice positive results like weight loss, better sleep, and improved mental clarity. This momentum can be seductive, causing them to stay comfortable with their new fasting lifestyle. But here's the challenge: The more someone stays on this schedule, the more hormetic stress dissipates, and hence fewer benefits result. In order to get the advantages of hormetic stress again, the lengths of the fasts have to be varied. Moving in and out of different lengths of fasts creates a continual hormetic stress on your cells, lovingly encouraging them to become metabolically stronger.

Heals your mitochondria

Metabolic switching is magic to your mitochondria. Often referred to as the powerhouses of your cells, your mitochondria perform two key functions: They provide you with energy and detox your cells. They take in glucose and nutrients from the foods you eat and turn them into adenosine triphosphate, or ATP, the biochemical name for energy. Every function of your body needs ATP to work properly. Without a proper surplus of ATP you will feel depleted, run-down, and stuck with your health.

Some of the hardest-working parts of your body have the densest amounts of mitochondria: your heart, liver, brain, eyes, and muscles. There can be several indications that your mitochondria are struggling. You may notice less muscle power in your workouts, you might find yourself sleepy often or chronically fatigued, your brain may be foggy and you have trouble concentrating, or you may struggle to go without food.

We are seeing that the mitochondria are indicators of our health. For years, chronic disease was blamed on unfortunate genetics. Recent discoveries from researchers like Thomas Seyfried, author of *Cancer as a Metabolic Disease*, have challenged this theory, stating that it's not our genetics that cause disease but rather malfunctioning mitochondria. Expanding upon the notable work of Otto War-burg, Nobel Prize winner for his research on the acidic changes that happen within cancer cells, Dr. Seyfried brought to light that disease begins in the mitochondria.[1] Once the mitochondria malfunction, disease can ensue inside the cell. Dr. Seyfried's research opened the door for other studies to follow looking at the mitochondrial changes that happen in a multitude of chronic diseases.

Metabolic switching has a positive impact on these mitochondria, which use both glucose and ketones for fuel.

When you eat, these little miracle machines take in the glucose that enters your cells and turns it into energy. When you fast, you make ketones that also get gobbled up by your mitochondria to be used for energy. When your mitochondria are sick, they become less efficient at using glucose, often leaving you tired after a meal. Periodic switching into different fasted states creates ketones that will repair your mitochondria and make them more capable of using glucose to your benefit.

Detoxing is the second critical job your mitochondria performs for you. It does this in two ways—it produces glutathione and controls methylation. Glutathione is your master antioxidant, credited with reducing oxidative stress, lowering cellular inflammation, improving insulin sensitivity, regenerating skin, helping with conditions like psoriasis and diseases such as Parkinson's, and having an overall positive effect on cardiovascular health. Methylation is a complex cellular process that can be simply explained as the pathway in which your cells push toxins out. When your mitochondria are healthy, they turn on methylation and swiftly escort toxins out of your cells. When your mitochondria are damaged, you will be low in glutathione, not methylating properly and therefore allowing toxins to stay stuck inside, leading to inflammation, damaged cell parts, and in some cases allowing disease genes to be triggered.

As you learn to metabolically switch, you begin to heal these mitochondria and restore cellular health.

Regenerates neurons in your brain

Every thought you think, memory you have, or emotion you feel travels across the trillions of your brain's neurons. If these neurons degenerate, you will see changes in your mental cognition, plain and simple. This may look like you are in the middle of a conversation and forget what you were saying or you walk into a room in your house and can't remember why you did so. Degenerating neurons may also feel like you struggle to hold on to new information when it's presented to you.

Neurons get impaired by poor diet, toxins like heavy metals, and lack of use. The most notorious example of what can result from neurodegeneration is Alzheimer's disease.

When you put yourself in a fasted state, you not only repair these malfunctioning neurons but you also encourage the growth of new neurons. When you eat foods that are rich in good fats, amino acids, vitamins, and minerals, you power up those neurons so they function at their best. It's flipping the metabolic switch between fasting and fed states that repairs the neurons in your brain best. Many women notice that the longer they practice the art of metabolic switching, the more vibrant they feel. Countless times I have heard fasting women in their 50s say they have more energy and better mental clarity than they did in their 30s.

Year after year you will notice that your body gets healthier because you are taking advantage of the four healing principles that metabolic switching provides. Now that you understand the underlying healing mechanisms that occur when you switch in and out of your two energy systems, let's look at what specific conditions metabolic switching works best for. Although your body will always thrive with this type of switching, there are seven very specific times when you will find moving in and out of these two healing metabolic states to be the miracle cure you've been searching for.

- Slows the aging clock
- Offers lasting weight loss
- Powers up memory
- Balances the gut
- Keeps away cancer
- Mobilizes toxins
- Alleviates autoimmune conditions

Turns back the clock (or at least slows the aging clock)

Although aging is inevitable, the speed at which you age is not. The key to slowing down the aging process is to ensure that you give your cells all the necessary resources they need to stay working at their best. Remember, healthy cells will replicate into more healthy cells. The name of the aging game is to keep your cells optimally healthy. It turns out that providing your cells some good old-fashioned hormetic stress keeps them strong. Routinely dipping into longer fasted states provides just the right amount of stress to force them to adapt.

Once again, the research on hormetic stress, fasting, and anti-aging is convincing. One form of fasting called alternate-day fasting increases the expression of an anti-aging gene known as SIRT1.[2] When activated, this gene is a key regulator of many cellular defenses that will allow for survival in response to stress. This gene also protects against disease processes that can form inside your cells. It has been reported that as little as three weeks of alternate-day fasting can significantly increase the expression of this gene, slowing down the aging process in your body. Pretty cool, right?

Offers lasting weight loss

Every diet you go on will continue to fail you if it doesn't provide the opportunity to move in and out of your two metabolic states—sugar burner and fat burner. Flipping your metabolic switch into fat-burning mode is the most efficient way to get your body to go after that excess glucose it has packed away for a rainy day. Fasting is that rainy day. You have to flip that metabolic switch to get lasting weight-loss results. In fact, there is growing scientific evidence that obese individuals' ability to switch over to fat-burning mode is impaired, and once they restore metabolic flexibility they can begin to lose weight.[3]

When you eat, which raises your blood glucose levels, your cells will burn energy from that food you just ingested. When you fast, you flip your metabolic switch and start making energy from burning fat. Where trendy diets fall short is that they work only with your sugar-burner system. If you change what you eat but not the timing of your food intake, you leave out the fat-burning energy system.

When you are looking for lasting weight loss, it's important to realize that you need to train your body to find the extra sugar it has stored away in your body. As you read earlier, your body likes to store extra sugar in three main places: fat, liver, and muscles. If you have been eating poorly for years, you most likely have built up a lot of sugar in those places. When you exercise, you force the release of the stored sugar from your muscles. But how do you get to the stored sugar in your fat and liver? By fasting. The longer you stay in a fasted state, the more the body will access this stored sugar. If you finish your dinner at 6 P.M. and don't eat until 11 A.M. the next day, you have given your body 17 hours to go after all of that stored sugar. Once you eat, you switch back to your sugar-burner system. The more times you move into the fasted state, the more you will force your body to release the excess sugar.

Powers up memory

Fifty percent of your brain runs on glucose, while the other 50 percent is fueled by ketones. If you have never fasted long enough to make ketones, you have been depriving your brain of half of the fuel source it requires.

Remember how your body makes ketones when you fast? Once your brain senses the presence of ketones, it will increase a powerful neurochemical called brain-derived neurotrophic factor, or BDNF for short. This neurochemical is like Miracle-Gro for your brain. BDNF stimulates the production of new neurons, giving your brain more resources to hold on to information. The surge in ketones also stimulates the production of GABA, a calming neurotransmitter. When these two neurochemicals are present, you are in the optimal state for learning. When the brain is calm, focused, and equipped with new neurons, you will retain information in a way you may have never experienced before.

Many fasters feel so productive in the fasted state that they want to stay there throughout their day, but as blissful as it sounds to have a surge of ketones improving your mental cognition, your brain is fueled 50 percent by ketones and 50 percent by glucose. So as much as we love ketones, eventually you'll need to switch back to your sugar-burner system to fuel your brain. It's the moving in and out of both energy systems that provides the brain with all the necessary fuel it needs to perform at its best.

Balances the gut

Fasting heals the gut. Research proves this. But many of the positive changes that happen to your gut microbiome stop when you eat. So does this mean that microbiome changes are only temporary? Absolutely not! When you break your fast with food that feeds your microbiome, you will continue to heal your gut. (I have dedicated all of Chapter 9, How to Break a Fast, to teach you exactly how to do that.)

There is a term that is often used when speaking of your gut microbiome: It's called your *gut terrain*. This refers to the environment in which the good gut bacteria can grow. You can change the terrain of your gut microbiome with fasting. This allows the mucosal lining of your gut to digest your foods more efficiently and make key neurotransmitters, like serotonin, that keep you happy. The growth of that good bacteria will continue when you eat if you feed them foods rich in polyphenols, probiotics, and prebiotics. Food will fuel those bacteria so that they can make neurotransmitters, support a healthy immune system, and provide you with necessary vitamins and minerals. Metabolically switching in and out of fasting and fed states will create the greatest impact on your gut microbiome. My clinical experience has taught me that this is the most effective way to heal any gut challenge you may be experiencing.

Keeps away cancer

Your mitochondria need ketones to heal. You can't stay in a constant state of sugar burning to heal your mitochondria. Yes, there are foods that nourish your mitochondria. Because of their unique nutrient content, among the most powerful foods that can positively impact your mitochondria are organ meats. A diet rich in vegetables coming from a wide variety of colors also gives your mitochondria the nutrients it needs to power up. But ketones heal the mitochondria best. Metabolic switching allows you to heal your mitochondria with both nutrients and ketones. Dr. Nasha Winters, author of *The Metabolic Approach to Cancer*, describes one of the early signs that your cells are becoming metabolically inflexible as when you get "hangry," especially if it has been only a few hours since you last ate. This is a telltale sign that your cells are not making that switch over to fat burning. Healthy mitochondria will easily adapt to declining glucose levels while waiting for the ketone surge. This metabolic switch will feel effortless, allowing you to go longer without food while it takes time for the liver to supply ketones. Unhealthy mitochondria, on the other hand, will struggle while waiting for that switch. Knowing that cancer begins with dysfunctional mitochondria, this makes metabolic switching an art that every woman who has had cancer or does not want cancer needs to learn. Remember the study that proved women who fasted 13 hours every day after conventional breast cancer treatment had a 64 percent less chance of recurrence of cancer? This result most likely happened because their 13-hour fasting window allowed them to repair the dysfunctional mitochondria that started the cancer in the first place. No doubt if they paired that 13-hour fast with good nutritious food, that chance of recurrence would most likely go down even more.

Mobilizes toxins

Fasting can move toxins out of your cells for excretion. This toxic release happens most often when you move in and out of

72

fasts that are longer than 17 hours. Remember that 17 hours of fasting activates autophagy. This trigger is like turning on the doctor inside each cell. That cellular doctor will decide if it can clean up that cell or if it needs to die. When cells are deemed too damaged and cellular death occurs, the toxins within the cells will enter your bloodstream to exit. It is at this point that all your detox organs will move into action to ensure those toxins leave your system. In the fasting world, we often refer to these organs as your detox pathways: your liver, gallbladder, gut, kidneys, and lymphatic system.

The more you metabolically switch using longer fasts, the more you may become aware that your detox pathways may be congested. We refer to these as closed pathways; symptoms of closed pathways include:

- Rashes
- Brain fog
- Feeling bloated
- Diarrhea
- Constipation
- Low energy

If you experience any of these symptoms, the first thing I want you to realize is it's common. I have seen some fasters who think that fasting is not working for them when these symptoms appear. Nothing is further from the truth! It's absolutely working. You just need to work on opening up those pathways so that your body can effortlessly remove those toxins without you even noticing. (In Chapter 10, Hacks That Make Fasting Effortless, I will show you specific protocols that work best for opening up your detox pathways.)

Alleviates autoimmune conditions

Autoimmune conditions happen for three very specific reasons: a damaged gut, an overload of toxins, and genetic predisposition. Metabolic switching can greatly help all three. It has been said that upward of 70 percent of your immune system is in your gut. Because of this, with any autoimmune condition you will have to repair the gut. Hopefully now you are seeing that metabolically switching is one of the most effective ways to repair your gut. Healing your mitochondria will also greatly improve an autoimmune condition. Remember, your mitochondria support your cell's ability to detox. When you heal your mitochondria, not only will they power up more of your detox antioxidant glutathione but your cells will become more proficient at moving toxins out of the cell. Once the mitochondria are functioning at their best and detox pathways are open, genes can be turned off. This is the basis of epigenetics. Our lifestyle influences genes that get turned on, and it also influences genes that get turned off.

A few years ago, I helped a 57-year-old woman named Nancy who had multiple autoimmune conditions stacking up. She not only had been diagnosed with Hashimoto's thyroiditis, but her body was attacking her mitochondria, giving her excessive levels of mitochondrial antibodies. (Antibodies are specialized cells of your immune system that are preprogrammed to attack not only certain pathogens that enter your body but anything that it identifies as a foreign invader.) With autoimmune conditions these antibodies often attack healthy tissue. If your body were attacking both your thyroid and your mitochondria, you would feel pretty horrible. That's exactly how Nancy felt. Extremely low in energy, suffering with poor mental clarity, and living with many unrelenting symptoms like chronic pain, Nancy was struggling to function in her day-to-day life. Her health was rapidly declining. She had been in and out of multiple doctors' offices with misdiagnoses, fancy medications to take, and lots of advice that told her she just had to live with it. Refusing to accept that treatment plan, Nancy reached out to me to see what she could do to take matters into her own hands. Although it took time to get Nancy's health back on track, unwinding her autoimmune condition wasn't as complex as one might think. Applying the principles of healing autoimmune conditions, I taught her how to move in and out of different food and fasting variations to help heal her gut and repair the damaged mitochondria that infiltrated her body. Over the course of a year, she tried out all six different-length fasts and several different food styles. We then moved on to detoxing her, identifying all the environmental toxins and heavy metals that were possibly building up in her body and causing her immune system to attack itself. The results Nancy experienced were downright miraculous. Within a year's time, her mitochondrial antibodies were cut in half and her thyroid antibodies had disappeared. Within two years of her healing journey, her antibodies had all returned to normal and her doctors were blown away that she showed no lingering signs of any autoimmune conditions. Metabolic switching combined with detox is magic for autoimmune conditions.

When you train your body to go in and out of fed and fasted states, you create a healing response in the body like no other. This is phenomenal news for women. We can lose weight, build muscle, balance hormones, power up our brains, repair our guts, slow down aging, and overcome an autoimmune condition all by just applying the fundamentals of metabolic switching to our lives. Now when we time that switching to your menstrual cycle—look out! You will discover a level of health you may have never thought possible.

That's what happened to a patient of mine named Carrie, who came to me asking for help to lower her BMI. At 32 she had hit a wall with her health, struggling with fertility issues and weight-loss resistance, and her ob-gyn pointed out that her BMI was too high, which could be contributing to her challenges to conceive a baby. Losing some weight might improve her chances of pregnancy. Repetitively failing at weight-loss diets was something Carrie knew quite well, so when her doctor told her dropping weight was her only solution to getting pregnant, she fell into a deep depression. She wasn't overweight because she overate. In fact, her diet was pretty good. She didn't lack willpower or discipline. Every diet Carrie ever tried, she followed to a tee. So what was she missing?

Enter metabolic switching. I started Carrie on a protocol of different-length fasts and types of food, that allowed her to metabolically switch. I showed her how to time that switch to her menstrual cycles, supporting her hormonal ebbs and flows. With a clear metabolic switch mapped out, I instructed Carrie to follow this routine for 90 days and check back in with me. Within a month I received a phone call from her. Not only did she lose 10 pounds in the first month of this new regime, but she was pregnant. This is the power of learning to metabolically switch to your menstrual cycle.

Now that you have a strong foundational understanding of the science behind fasting and why you thrive with metabolic switching, I am excited to show you how to take these concepts and map them to your hormonal needs. It's time to officially learn how to fast like a girl!

CHAPTER 4

Fasting a Woman's Way

Bridget—a type-A high-tech executive—had a very demanding career, two active teenage girls, and an overscheduled life that never quite allowed her to relax. Stress was something that Bridget knew all too well. An avid runner, exercise was her drug of choice. She ran to keep her weight down, calm her brain, and help deal with her frantic pace of life. When she turned 40, she felt invincible. By 42, however, she had turned into a hot mess. The first major symptom Bridget noticed was that she started gaining weight for no particular reason, especially around her midsection. Relying on her old weight-loss tricks, she tried eating less and exercising more, but that stubborn belly fat wouldn't budge. The more she tried to exercise her way out of her new health hurdles, the more her injuries piled up. Pulled calf muscles, episodic lower back problems, and old rotator cuff injuries kept rearing their ugly heads. This new reality was making it incredibly difficult to work out. Without running as a weight-loss and stress-management tool, Bridget fell into a deep depression. Looking for a new lifestyle tool to replace exercise, Bridget heard from a friend that she should try intermittent fasting. Being the overachiever that she was, Bridget wanted to learn everything she could about how she could master fasting. She started by skipping breakfast and putting MCT oil in her coffee to see if she could fast a little longer. Pretty quickly she noticed that she was getting the hang of fasting and was loving the results. Soon she became obsessed with fasting, feeling better and better the more time she spent in a fasted state. Her mental clarity, energy, and calmness was at an all-time high. She also noticed that fasting freed up her time, killed her hunger, and gave her the same fitness results that running had. She was in love with this new fasting lifestyle!

About six months in, however, Bridget started having some adverse symptoms. The first was heart palpitations. She would be sitting at her desk in the middle of the day and her heart would start racing. Knowing that her life was full of all kinds of stressors, her first thought was that her overscheduled life was finally catching up with her. The racing heart quickly turned into anxiety. She would have panic attacks in the middle of the day for no apparent reason. She couldn't figure out what triggered these attacks or, worse yet, how to stop them. Then her sleep went sideways. She couldn't get her body to relax enough to fall asleep and would often wake up at two in the morning struggling to get back to sleep. Then one morning in the shower, she noticed clumps of her hair falling out. This continued for weeks until she had visible bald spots. Concerned, she went to her doctor, who ran extensive blood work that all came back normal. Her doctor asked about her diet, and Bridget told her about her fasting regimen. To her surprise, her doctor advised her to stop, pointing out that fasting wasn't good for women. This crushed Bridget—she felt stuck, depressed, and out of answers.

Luckily, her friend recommended she watch my YouTube videos on how women should fast. She was surprised to hear that there is more to fasting than just skipping meals and that women should approach fasting differently than men, varying it according to their monthly hormone fluctuations. Perhaps fasting wasn't the problem, she thought, it's that she wasn't fasting like a girl. She hadn't been varying her fasts to match the ebbs and flows of her hormones. This new information gave Bridget hope. She immediately changed her fasting regime to coordinate to her monthly hormonal needs, and within one month her hair stopped falling out, the anxiety and panic attacks went away, and she began sleeping soundly again.

Your menstrual cycle is truly a miraculous symphony of neurochemical responses that work in perfect harmony for your reproductive benefit. If up until now you have looked at your menstrual cycle as just a bothersome event, I encourage you to rethink the magic that is happening in you every month. Our menstrual cycles are rarely discussed, evaluated, or looked at as a health priority. This ignorance affects us in so many ways, but ultimately it leads us to not fully appreciate how our lifestyle can influence the intricate design of this hormonal system. Without a proper understanding of our menstrual cycles, our hormones suffer, which means our whole body suffers. When you learn to fast like a girl, you bring synergy back to these beautiful neurochemicals that serve you so well.

I know this because like Bridget, I found out the hard way. When I hit 40 and my hormones started to go on a wild ride through perimenopause, I realized that although I understood the mechanics behind my menstrual cycle, I didn't fully grasp how the ebbs and flows of my hormones affected my moods, productivity, sleep, and even my motivations, nor did I know how to match my lifestyle to my monthly hormonal shift. Most of us haven't been taught how to time our lifestyle habits to our hormones. In fact, most women don't know what hormones are coming or going in a 28-day period. This is a massive problem and is contributing to too many hormonal imbalances for women. Education around how to time everything from our foods, exercise, social calendars, and fasting behaviors needs to start at puberty. Why aren't we teaching girls these things? Once you get the hang of the hormones that are coming and going throughout your menstrual cycle, you will begin to see that timing your lifestyle to maximize your hormonal performance will have you feeling like the rock star you were born to be.

The first thing to know about your monthly menstrual cycle is that yours is unique. All women have different-length cycles. Most women's cycles last around 28 days; some are shorter, while others can go as long as 30-plus days. The second thing to know about your menstrual cycle is that hormones rise and fall throughout. They don't stay at a consistent level all month long. There is an ebb and flow to them. This is important to know because you will feel different emotionally and physically at different times of the month because of this rise and fall.

Perhaps the most complex part of hormones is that they are constant moving targets. As you will see when I map out the hormonal hierarchy for you, each hormone greatly influences the performance of the next hormone. If one hormone lags, the whole team can fall apart. Getting to know the effects that each of these hormones have on your moods, sleep, motivations, energy, appetite, and ability to fast will be life changing.

The fun part about fasting like a girl is that you are about to get to know these hormones well. I'm going to introduce you to the primary hormones of your menstrual cycle and how they rise and fall throughout the month. (If you currently don't have a cycle, don't dismiss this next section, as I want you to get to know the influence these hormones have on your life. In Part III, I will show you how to amplify these hormones even if your cycle is irregular or no longer age appropriate.)

YOUR MENSTRUAL CYCLE

Days 1–10

At the beginning of your menstrual cycle, on day one, your major sex hormones—estrogen, testosterone, and progesterone—are at their lowest levels. Within a few days after your cycle has started, your hypothalamus, the part of your brain responsible for coordinating hormone production, begins to pulse the hormones you need for your ovaries to release an egg. This pulsing of key hormones causes estrogen to slowly build within you until it reaches its peak somewhere mid-ovulation (around day 13).

As your estrogen builds, you will notice several things happen to you physically and mentally. First, estrogen contributes to the production of collagen, which keeps your skin young and supple. This boost in collagen also makes your bones strong and ligaments more elastic, making you less injury prone, especially when pushing your workouts to new levels. At menopause estrogen drops, and that's when we start to see the dreaded wrinkles and we become more prone to injury.

Estrogen also puts you in a good mood, gives you clarity of thought, enhances your communication skills, and makes you feel more optimistic about life. How? Estrogen is a precursor to serotonin, dopamine, and noradrenaline—the neurotransmitters that keep you calm, happy, and feeling satisfied. Estrogen also calms the fear centers of your brain. Research published in *Biological Psychiatry* revealed that when a woman is low in estrogen she is more vulnerable to traumas, while high levels of estrogen can partially protect a woman from emotional disturbances.[1] As your estrogen is building in this part of your menstrual cycle, you may find yourself with a better outlook on life and with the ability to handle stressful events with more ease. For example, a breakup with a significant other may be more emotionally challenging for you if it happens when estrogen is low. That's how impactful these hormones can be!

Days 11–15

This is known as your ovulation period. Although all the three sex hormones come into play at this time, it's estrogen and testosterone that will influence you the most during this five-day period. The physical and mental benefits of estrogen continue to build, while the addition of testosterone can make you feel powerful and strong during this five-day window. Between the surge in estrogen enhancing your mental clarity and moods and testosterone giving you motivation, drive, and energy, this is a great time to start a new project, lean in to a difficult task, or add a few more things to your daily to-do list. It's a great time to ask for a raise, take on a tough conversation, or launch a new business. Testosterone also helps you build muscle, so increasing your strength-training workouts during this time may yield more of a muscle-building response.

Days 16–18

This is the time when all of your hormones dip. You will feel very much like you do the first week of your cycle, with one major exception: Instead of your body preparing to make estrogen, your body ramps up to make progesterone. You may feel supercharged during ovulation, but as you enter this stage you may experience a dip in energy and mental clarity.

Day 19—Bleed

This is the moment your body produces progesterone, the hormone that calms you and tells you everything is going to be okay. During this time of your cycle, you will often feel less aggressive, less irritable, and more like you want to sit on the couch and chill than go out and socialize. Progesterone's job is to prepare your uterine lining for a fertilized egg to implant post ovulation. Depending on when you ovulate, your progesterone levels usually hit their peak six to eight days after ovulation. This means that if an egg released on day 14 of your cycle, your progesterone levels will be their highest around day 19.

When you start building a fasting lifestyle, this last stage is the most important to be mindful of because progesterone is very influenced by cortisol. If estrogen thrives when insulin is low, progesterone thrives when cortisol is low. There is a precursor steroid hormone called DHEA that you need to make progesterone. If during this phase of your monthly cycle your cortisol spikes too much, you won't have enough DHEA to make progesterone. This scenario is common, and can lead to missed cycles, days of spotting, increased irritability, and trouble sleeping. How many years as women have we complained about our premenstrual symptoms, when in reality it's a simple function of not giving our body the right scenarios to make progesterone.

There are many situations in our life that raise cortisol and cause progesterone to plummet. Of course, there are the unavoidable traumas that happen throughout our lives, and since the larger stressors tend to happen unexpectedly, we can only course-correct and bring our cortisol levels down as we move through those moments. But then we have other mild stressors that happen on a more regular basis that we can prepare for and make sure don't cause a dip in progesterone. These include good stressors like exercise and fasting. Both of those health habits cause mild, temporary rises in cortisol that although ultimately support your body to adapt and build itself stronger, can cause your progesterone levels to fall. I encourage you to not fast the week before your period, as even minor healthy spikes of cortisol can tank your progesterone. This is especially important for perimenopausal women, who still may have a cycle but also have age-appropriate declining progesterone levels.

The other aspect of progesterone that you will want to be aware of as you build a fasting lifestyle is the influence glucose and insulin have over this miraculous calming hormone. Estrogen and progesterone, although both sex hormones, really require different behaviors from us. Estrogen doesn't seem as influenced by cortisol but really suffers when glucose and insulin are high. Progesterone suffers when cortisol is high but actually requires more glucose in your bloodstream to fully develop to the levels that are necessary for your period to start. If you fast during this time or restrict carbohydrates, you may not give progesterone the fuel it needs. I will go into more detail on this in Chapter 6.

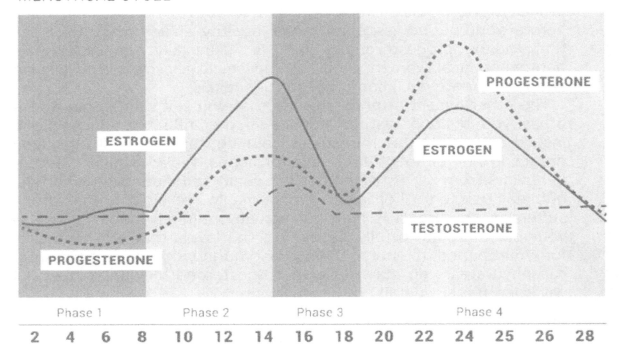

WHY WE NEED TO FAST DIFFERENTLY

Can you see how complex and brilliantly designed your body is? This is a big overarching reason that we need to fast differently. Men are hormonally simpler. They have a 24-hour hormone cycle with one main hormone—testosterone—moving in and out of their bodies every 15 minutes. Men don't have the ebbs and flows of estrogen and progesterone to contend with. Whether we actively have a menstrual cycle or not, we must take into consideration all three of our major hormones—estrogen, progesterone, and testosterone—that rise and fall monthly and throughout our menopausal journey. Where a man can fast in a similar fashion every day of the month, we women need to pay attention to four distinct times within our monthly cycle. And we also need to take a look into three important and uniquely female features as we fast differently than men:

- The power of our hormonal hierarchy
- Fluctuations in our sex hormones
- The impact of our toxic loads

The Power of Our Hormonal Hierarchy

This first is a principle called the hormonal hierarchy. Here's how it works: The hormone oxytocin can calm cortisol. Cortisol spikes will cause increases in insulin, and surges in insulin have a direct effect over your sex hormones estrogen, progesterone, and testosterone. When we fast, we have to pay close attention to how these hormones all impact each other.

How does this work? You have two areas in your brain—the hypothalamus and pituitary—that balance all the hormones in your body. The hypothalamus receives hormonal information from your endocrine organs and uses that info to tell the pituitary gland what hormones it needs to make. The pituitary gland then takes that instruction and sends a hormonal signal back to your endocrine organ to signal what hormones are still needed. It is like an air traffic control tower that scans the incoming flights and coordinates the landing of thousands of planes. Once the plane lands, the signal gets back to the tower that it's safely arrived at the gate.

Here is where the hierarchy comes into play. Much like the air traffic control tower has to make a decision about the order of flights that land, your hypothalamus does the same as it is receiving thousands of hormonal signals. It must decide which hormones your body needs more of and which ones it should turn off. When the hypothalamus receives cortisol signals from your adrenal glands, it tells the pituitary there is a crisis at hand. The pituitary modulates glucose metabolism by sending a signal to the pancreas to get ready because glucose is about to be released by the tissues. The pancreas responds by revving up insulin.

Insulin

When insulin surges in the body, that signal goes back up to the hypothalamus, which tells the pituitary to shut off production of estrogen and progesterone because the crisis is still brewing. From an evolutionary standpoint, there is no need to procreate when a crisis is underway, so these sex hormones become unnecessary. Are you starting to see how this hierarchy works? Cortisol starts the whole cascade of hormonal responses. Here is where this hierarchy gets fun. If you know stress is high, causing insulin and sex hormone imbalances, then you want to focus first on the top of the hormonal chain. Remember which hormone is at the top of the hormonal chain? Oxytocin. The minute the brain gets the oxytocin signal, it turns off cortisol, leading to better glucose management, a reduction in insulin, and a rebalancing of sex hormones. One key hormone brings the whole system back into balance.

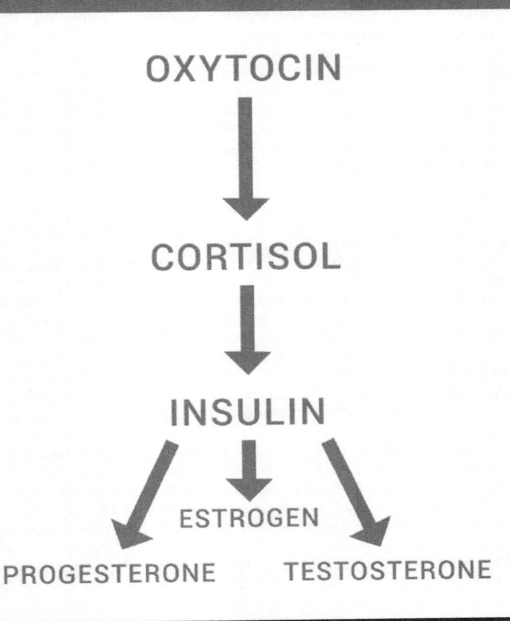

All too often I watch women try to balance their sex hormones without realizing that they need to be insulin sensitive and have minimal spikes in cortisol. If a woman is under chronic amounts of stress mixed with being insulin resistant, balancing her sex hormones will be a dead-end street. To truly get to the root cause of any sex hormone challenge, you need to take this whole hierarchy into consideration. I watch women struggle with classic hormonal imbalances like infertility, PCOS, or unruly menopause symptoms. Many times the treatment they are using to overcome these challenges is addressing only one piece of this hierarchy. When a woman discovers tools to help balance stress, insulin, and her sex hormones, she will finally see a change in these conditions.

Cortisol

Getting stress under control is no doubt easier said than done. For years, I personally struggled with the mental and physical effects of too much cortisol surging through me. Good friends would tell me to slow down and lean in to more self-care. This was not an easy request. After reading *Rushing Woman's Syndrome*, in which Dr. Weaver describes in exquisite detail the impact cortisol has on a woman's body, I began to understand at a deeper level the negative physiological consequence cortisol was having on my hormonal health. This motivated me to change my stressful ways. Most likely you have also had moments when cortisol has hijacked your hormonal health and you too have witnessed this hierarchy at play.

Often women see the most hormonal dysfunction during or after times of chronic stress. When stress levels go up, cortisol levels spike. A surge of cortisol signals to your body to elevate your blood sugar. This is your classic fight-or-flight response. Your body prepares as if it needs to run away from a tiger that's chasing you, releasing stored sugar to send to your muscles quickly so you can act. Your body adapts to this new surge in blood sugar by telling your pancreas to make more insulin. If you are trying to lose weight, this chemical reaction can really work against you. Cortisol can raise insulin as much as a piece of cake can. This can make it difficult to lose weight when you are living a high-stress life. This increased insulin initiated by cortisol spikes sets you up to fail at any diet, fast, or nutrition change you are trying to make. But the damage from cortisol doesn't stop there. Continued cortisol spikes signaling insulin deplete your sex hormone production. Combine chronic stress with eating the classic Western diet and you will find balancing estrogen, progesterone, and testosterone difficult.

Can you see why your health goals have eluded you in times of stress? Cortisol is the bully in the play yard that makes sure no other hormones can play. Depressing, right? Well, here is the good news. Fasting like a girl can not only help you unwind the negative effects cortisol plays on your body; it can also help improve production of neurotransmitters that calm you, helping you combat stress with more grace.

Also, keep in mind that there is one key hormone that will stop cortisol in its tracks and break this chronic stress cycle. At the top of the hierarchy sits one powerful hormone that can balance all the other hormones that sit below. It's oxytocin.

Oxytocin

When you make oxytocin, your cortisol levels will drop, balancing out your insulin levels and leading to better sex hormone production. You might know oxytocin as the love hormone. Getting more of this hormone is super fun! You get a dose of oxytocin from hugging, talking with your best friend, laughing, petting your dog, holding a baby saying, "I love you," being in a state of gratitude, snuggling, sex, masturbation, meditation, yoga, massage, and deep, meaningful conversations with people. Don't dismiss these activities as being frivolous uses of your time. As a woman, you need lots of oxytocin. More so than your male counterparts. Most important, oxytocin is at the top of the hierarchy, so it means it has the power to balance all of your other hormones. Oxytocin has a direct effect on the hypothalamus of your brain. When oxytocin is on the scene, it tells your brain that you are safe and loved and the crisis is over. The brain responds by ceasing the production of cortisol. How awesome is that?! Your health will benefit greatly from getting daily doses of oxytocin.

FLUCTUATIONS OF OUR SEX HORMONES

Have you ever had one of those days when you felt unusually hungry for no particular reason? If you have been in the habit of counting calories, this can be the day you beat yourself up for not being able to stick to your diet. Or what about the carbohydrate cravings that kick in out of the blue? Do you find yourself reaching for a cookie in that moment only to end up eating the whole box? I'm pretty sure every woman has gone through appetite and craving swings within a month, never linking those cravings to the changes in her monthly hormones. We shame ourselves when we eat foods that our bodies crave but our minds tell us we shouldn't eat. What if the foods you choose are not within your mental control? What if they are being orchestrated by your hormones?

For the sake of this conversation, what is pivotal to understand is that in a one-month cycle there will be times that fasting will feel effortless and times when fasting will be difficult. This is not because you are undisciplined. This happens because each sex hormone responds differently to two major hormones—insulin and cortisol.

Estrogen

Estrogen loves when you fast. The longer the fast, the better. In the beginning of your cycle when estrogen is building, any of the six fasting lengths will magnify her glory. Here's why. Estrogen thrives when insulin is low. Estrogen and insulin have a beautiful dance they do together. When insulin goes high-estrogen goes low, and vice versa. Just ask any menopausal woman: As she moved through her menopausal years, she likely struggled to keep weight off. The wild ride of estrogen dramatically going up and down during her perimenopause years contributes to more insulin resistance. The cycling woman experiences the negative effects of high insulin on her estrogen levels as well. If insulin stays consistently high, it alters the pituitary gland, the part of the brain that signals estrogen to be released from your ovaries. This is a common scenario for women who struggle with infertility: high insulin and little estrogen production leading to impaired ovulation.

Because of fasting's ability to decrease insulin, all six fasts work well when your body is making estrogen. In Chapter 8 I will introduce you to a tool called the Fasting Cycle that will show you exactly how to time your longer fasts to the best days in your cycle. For now, know that whenever estrogen is low your fasts will feel much easier.

Testosterone

The effect of fasting on testosterone production is an interesting one. Studies show that daily intermittent fasting can greatly increase a man's testosterone, but no female studies have been done. In cases like this we have to make assumptions and combine them with clinical experience. My clinical experience has shown me that when testosterone comes in during ovulation, intermittent fasting no longer than 15 hours is best. The ovulation window is when you have both estrogen and testosterone surging at full force with a tiny bit of progesterone. Moderate-level fasting of 15 hours at this time is perfect, but not any longer. This part of your monthly cycle is so spectacular because you see all three hormones showing up. This makes you unusually powerful. You will feel your best when estrogen, testosterone, and progesterone are balanced during ovulation. Cortisol can greatly decrease both testosterone and progesterone, so this would not be the time to launch into a three-day water fast.

Progesterone

Perhaps the most important time to avoid fasting during your monthly cycle is the week before your period. This is when your body is making progesterone. Two qualities of progesterone that make fasting a bad option—its susceptibility to both cortisol and glucose. First, progesterone declines when cortisol gets high. Any activity that raises cortisol will tank your progesterone levels. Second, progesterone prefers you keep glucose on the higher side. Any diet that keeps glucose low, like the ketogenic diet, will also negatively impact your progesterone levels. These two influences on progesterone make fasts of all lengths a terrible option the week before your cycle.

Your Thyroid Hormones

One set of hormones that I would be remiss in not pointing out are your thyroid hormones, because there is an important interplay between them and your sex hormones. When your sex hormones drop, it can trigger hypothyroidism, causing weight gain, hair loss, fatigue, and depression. Because women are 10 times more likely than men to get thyroid problems, I want to make sure you understand how your thyroid hormones work.

First, your thyroid needs five organs to work properly: brain, thyroid, liver, gut, and adrenals. Your brain, specifically the pituitary gland that sits at the base of the skull, will release TSH (thyroid stimulating hormone), which travels down to the thyroid and activates it to make a hormone called thyroxine, or T4. This hormone then travels to the liver and gut to get converted into another version of thyroid hormone called triiodothyronine, or T3. This version is bioactive, meaning that once it's converted to T3 your cells will welcome that hormone in and use it for metabolism. What's important to know about this cascade of thyroid hormone production is that it requires your brain, liver, and gut to be working at their best. Your cells also have to be in an optimal state, free from toxins and inflammation, in order to receive these hormones. Fasting can absolutely help with the healing of all the players involved with thyroid health. In Appendix C, I give you my favorite fasting protocols for improving thyroid function.

THE IMPACT OF OUR TOXIC LOADS

Toxins can affect hormones in two ways. First, a well-known fact is that exposure to chemicals in our environment known as endocrine disruptors dramatically impacts our hormone production. Of the hundreds of thousands of man-made chemicals that exist in our world, a thousand of them have been proven to be endocrine disruptors, which down the line can lead to chronic diseases like breast cancer and polycystic ovarian syndrome.

The second way that is not talked about often is the reverse happening. Huge swings in hormones, specifically estrogen and progesterone, cause the release of toxins stored in a variety of your tissues. Lead is stored in your bones, liver, and lungs. Mercury in your kidneys, liver, and brain. Environmental pollutants are stored in fat tissue. Aluminum in your prefrontal cortex of your brain. When estrogen and progesterone rise, it can trigger these toxins to be slowly released.

So here we are, the third characteristic of the female body: Our hormonal surges can cause stored toxins to be released from our tissues, especially during pregnancy. According to the CDC, lead stored in a woman's bones is released during pregnancy. Although during pregnancy is when estrogen and progesterone levels are at their highest, you still have surges of estrogen when you ovulate, and progesterone the week before your period. When these two hormones rise, stored toxins can be released.

Here's where the problem exists. If you are going into longer fasts that stimulate autophagy during the upswing moments of estrogen and progesterone, you may be getting a double dose of toxins released into your bloodstream. Remember, when you stimulate autophagy in a cell, sometimes the intelligence within the cell decides that cell is better off dying. In that cellular death, any toxin stored inside will be redistributed into your body, most commonly in your nervous tissue and fat. During your ovulation period, as estrogen comes surging in, heavy metals like lead can get released from your bones. If you are deep into a fast stimulating autophagy at that same moment, you might find that you have some severe detox symptoms. When hormones go high, fasting lengths should go low.

All too often I hear couples decide to embark upon their fasting journeys together. They quickly discover that they get drastically different results. Most often women experience detox reactions such as hair loss, fat accumulation, brain fog, or rashes. If a woman is stimulating autophagy while her hormones are coming in strong, she can get more symptoms than a man will. Testosterone doesn't cause the release of toxins like estrogen and progesterone do.

Fasting like a girl means finding your own unique path to fasting and minding these hormonal moments. Jude, a 45-year-old woman I coached years ago, wanted to know how to build herself a fasting lifestyle. Struggling with weight-loss resistance, anxiety, and low energy, she had tested high for mercury and lead, two heavy metals that are often passed down from mother to child that can contribute to the above symptoms. Before consulting with me she kept trying to fast at the same intensity and frequency as her husband. Fasting for him seemed effortless, and he was dropping weight very quickly. Yet Jude was actually *gaining* weight and feeling incredibly anxious when she fasted, especially during any fast that lasted more than 17 hours. When I first met with her, she was not aware that she needed to modify her fasting routine according to her monthly cycle. I amended Jude's fasts so that when estrogen was peaking during ovulation and progesterone was increasing the week before her period, she drastically shortened her fasts so as not to stimulate autophagy. This helped dramatically, and very quickly she started to drop weight, the anxiety greatly improved, and her energy felt limitless. These are the feelings you should have when you fast, but it's imperative that you watch the moments your hormones come surging in.

If you keep in mind these three principles as you build your fasting lifestyle, you'll appreciate all the upsides of fasting without any negative hormonal consequences like Bridget and Jude had. There are so many wonderful ways fasting can serve our physical and mental health, but we have to do it the way our bodies respond best.

Now that you have a solid understanding of your hormonal superpowers, let's put them to good use and customize a fasting lifestyle that yields the health results you deserve.

PART II

THE ART OF FASTING LIKE A GIRL

CHAPTER 5

Build a Fasting Lifestyle Unique to You

Out of the ashes of frustration from a one-size-fits-all healthcare system, a new concept has emerged called personalized health care, often referred to as functional medicine. The imperative word here is *functional*. How do you build a health program that keeps you functioning at your best? All too often when you are diagnosed with a condition, it becomes a box you get put in that labels you stuck with that condition. High blood pressure is a great example of this. For each person who receives this diagnosis, the root cause may be different. Yet conventional medicine gives the same solution to everyone with high blood pressure—medication. Frustrated with this generic approach, millions of people are flocking to functional medicine practitioners to discover why their personal health conditions began and what they can do to resolve their own health crisis.

Individualized health care is not a new approach to health: Our old pal Hippocrates was a strong proponent of personalizing his treatments. It has been well documented in more than 70 of his works that he believed in the individuality of disease. He advocated for giving different drugs for different patterns, evaluating factors such as a person's constitution, age, and physique, as well as the time of year to determine which drugs he would prescribe. It's this *holistic*—meaning the whole body—approach that many are waking up to. Even though a symptom may be common, the treatment must be unique to each individual body.

At the center of this personalized functional approach to health lives a concept called *n* of 1, commonly used in psychotherapy clinical trials with great success. Patients participating in *n*-of-1 trials are an active part of the treatment decision-making process. In this model of treatment, doctors collaborate with their patients to find the right healing path that's unique to them. This collaborative approach has been shown to improve health outcomes among patients with chronic illness.[1] It's been well documented that a patient who participates in an *n*-of-1 trial has a greater understanding and awareness of their condition and feels a greater sense of control when it comes to decisions about their health.[2] This personal empowerment approach works to heal not only your mind but also your body. This is the approach I want you to take with fasting.

Building a fasting lifestyle is a personal journey where you discover a path that works best *for you*. That means figuring out how to incorporate fasting into your life, no matter how busy that life is. Determining how long you want to be in a fasted state each day is a definite necessity and can be a whole lot of fun once you find your fasting rhythm. You can customize your fasting lengths according to your body's needs and what you may be trying to achieve. You can also customize your fasts when life events dictate changes to your regimen, such as vacations, social obligations, and work schedules. Most diets are rigid and hard to customize, often forcing you to modify your life to meet the demands of your new health plan, rather than the other way around. Let fasting work for you. To do that, let's consider what I call "the four pillars" as you start your journey.

FOUR PILLARS OF A FASTING LIFESTYLE

PILLAR #1-Identify Your Goals

What you are trying to accomplish with fasting is pivotal. I can't tell you the number of Q&A sessions I have done with my online community where someone asks me, "What fast is best for me?" I wish it were that simple! It all depends on what you are trying to achieve with your fasts. Because each of the six fasts I've outlined in this book has different healing effects, it's really important as you go to build a fasting lifestyle that is in line with what you want to achieve. Is it weight loss? Is it to have more energy? Just because I have laid out six different-length fasts doesn't mean you will necessarily want to do all six. Typically, I find women use fasting for three reasons: to lose weight, balance hormones, and/or overcome a specific condition.

Lose weight

As with many diets, it's very common for women to lose weight very differently than men as they build a fasting lifestyle. For example, men can start fasting 15 hours a day and drop 30 pounds within a month. Women typically don't lose weight as fast. I applaud couples who embark on lifestyle changes together, as it's much easier to do it with a partner, but when one loses quickly it often leaves the other feeling deflated.

The second thing to keep in mind when you go to fast as a woman is that you may need to lean in to longer fasts every once in a while. Like I mentioned before, throwing in a 36-hour fast can greatly accelerate weight-loss results, especially for women. Creating that deeper hormetic stress at the right time of your cycle can really turn the switch on your weight-loss results. Just make sure that you are doing it at the right time.

Balance hormones

Many women have found fasting to be an effective tool for regulating hormonal conditions like PCOS, infertility, and menopause symptoms. For these conditions, fasting like a girl really shines. When you start to regulate insulin, you may find that your sex hormones balance out naturally. Having said that, keep in mind that hormones are a bit of a moving target, so I have a few recommendations for you. First and foremost, be sure to follow the protocols for the conditions that I outline for you in Part III of this book.

The second thing to remember when your goal is to use fasting to balance hormones is to be patient. I have seen it take up to 90 days of fasting like a girl to find your fasting rhythm. Certain conditions resolve quickly when you start to use the concepts of metabolically switching to your hormonal advantage; others take time. I have found that the longer a hormonal imbalance has been with you, the more time it can take to resolve. But miracles can happen when you fast like a girl, so don't give up. With time and repetition, fasting will work for you.

When it comes to hormonal imbalances, you may want to get a urinary hormone test like the DUTCH test to know specifically which hormones are out of balance and how you can best go about mapping your fasts to fix those hormones. For example, if you know your estrogen levels are low you might want to do a longer fast in the first 15 days of your cycle, whereas if progesterone is low you want to make sure you're not fasting the week before your period.

Alleviate specific conditions

A lot of women want to use fasting to overcome challenges like an autoimmune condition, cancer diagnosis, diabetes, mood disorders, dementia, or Alzheimer's. Once again, fasting can dramatically improve these conditions, although each has its own specific protocols to follow (all laid out in Appendix C). Think of these protocols as fasting treatment plans. In my own clinical practice, I like to use fasting as my first go-to tool to help a patient. If you are suffering with any of the conditions I lay out for you, be sure to follow the associated protocol.

PILLAR #2-Vary Your Fasting Lengths

The goal with fasting is to learn a pattern that works for you and that you can maintain effortlessly as an ongoing health habit. When you first learn to fast, the most important step is to discover the best hours for you to skip food. My clinical observation has been that most people find their first fasting groove eating within an eight-hour window that goes from about 11 in the morning to 7 at night.

Once you have this base fasting time and length, your next step is to think how you might start to incorporate different-length fasts. We call this fasting variation, and it is a powerful way to make sure you never plateau with your fasting results. There are three reasons you want to vary your fasts: to avoid plateaus, to best honor your hormonal surges, and to give you flexibility.

Avoid plateaus

Because your body is programmed to always work to stay in balance, when you fast in the same way every day your body will begin to get comfortable. This can mean you stop getting results, just like with any diet or exercise program, when your body can hit plateaus. So variation is important. Small stressors force the body to adapt and build itself stronger; without those stressors the body becomes complacent. Varying your fasting lengths keeps your body guessing and gives it just enough of a hormetic stress to continuously work at its best.

Honor your hormonal surges

Women's bodies demand that we vary our fasts to match our hormones. If you follow the Fasting Cycle by varying your fasts to meet the influx of your hormones, you will find a natural rhythm that makes fasting feel effortless. We have a natural variation plan inherently built into us. It is when we don't tune in to this menstrual variation and map our fasts out accordingly that adverse fasting reactions happen. When you vary your fasts in accordance with your hormonal surges, you honor the needs of estrogen and progesterone. Estrogen will shine when you fast a little longer, while progesterone doesn't want you to fast too much.

There are two key times to alter your fasts: when your hormone levels peak at ovulation and the week before your period starts. Remember, when your sex hormones are at their highest—ovulation and the week before your period—your fasts should be shorter. When your hormone levels are low—when your cycle first starts and post ovulation—your fasts can be longer. You will see how this all plays out with the Fasting Cycle in Chapter 8.

A common indicator that a woman is not varying her fasts to best match her cycle is in the results she gets. Some women notice they start gaining weight, others will lose their periods, or old symptoms will creep back in. I have witnessed too many women fasting against the natural groove of their hormones, leading them down a path of unwanted symptoms. Keeping in mind that our bodies thrive on cycles will serve you well as you build your fasting lifestyle.

Be flexible

Any lifestyle tool that is too rigid and hard to follow will fail over time, no doubt about it. The beautiful part of varying your fasts is that you can fit it into the natural routine changes of your life. This flexibility sets you up for success.

We are talking vacation, holidays, times when a broken routine necessitates a change in fasting lengths. Say there is a big office holiday party—I suggest fasting all day and then letting yourself enjoy all of that great food with colleagues that night. If family is in town and they want to go out to breakfast? Maybe just don't fast at all that day. Or maybe you are on vacation. Who wants to deprive themselves of great food while away? Enjoy it. Once back home or back in your routine, you can hop right back on your more structured fasting regimen.

Flexibility is what makes building a fasting lifestyle so fun. You get to create it however it fits best into what life experiences are before you. This is a huge shortcoming of too many diets. If you are at home with a routine, that diet may be easy to follow. Once that routine changes or you are presented with a social gathering that doesn't have the food your diet requires, you are stuck with the difficult decision of what to eat. Fasting is freedom.

PILLAR #3-Vary Your Food Choices

Do you find yourself eating the same foods over and over again? For years, I would ask women this question, and the answer was the same: They do, indeed, eat the same 30-odd foods repeatedly. But repeat after me: Your feminine body thrives when you make new, unique, diverse food choices. Remember those diets you've been on that had you eating the same food every day? That's not serving your hormones or your gut. In the next section, I will walk you through the two food variations I recommend for women that will give you the variety your body needs to run optimally: ketobiotic and hormone feasting.

One reason we often choose the same foods is because of cravings. It's common to let your taste buds dictate your food choices. Cravings are often a hurdle that many women have trouble overcoming. If your brain keeps sending you signals that it wants foods that don't support your health, long-term health will always allude you. If this depresses you, don't let it. You can change your stubborn cravings by varying the foods you choose. With each new food you try, you feed new microbes. As these microbes thrive, they will send signals back to your brain telling it to crave new foods. Numerous studies are proving that your microbiome has a strong influence on your food preferences. For example, did you know that you have microbes in your gut that make you crave chocolate? Ask anyone who has been diagnosed with candida, a fungus that lives in the gut, and they will tell you that they have a ridiculous craving for sweets. This is because a fungus like candida will affect your food preferences by sending signals to your brain, telling your brain what it wants you to eat to stay alive. How insane is that?! If you succumb to these microbes' food preferences, eating the foods they demand over and over again, they will only get stronger. One of the benefits of varying both your fasts and foods is that over time you change the terrain in your gut and kill the critters. As these microbes die, so will your cravings. In my clinical practice, I have noticed that building a fasting lifestyle is more powerful for changing cravings than any other tool I have seen. And the research is proving this as well!

PILLAR #4-Surround Yourself with a Supportive Community

A large part of success to any diet regimen rests on having a support system who has your back. When you surround yourself with supportive people who are as excited for this new journey as you are, that positivity has a cascading effect. And remember, as women we are naturally built for community. Remember the hormonal hierarchy? All your hormones are greatly influenced by the queen hormone, oxytocin. When you are building a fasting lifestyle that influences insulin, you amplify your results by maximizing oxytocin. Connecting with others in community gives you a massive oxytocin burst. Honestly, I think this is one of the reasons the women in my online community get such amazing results. I have surrounded them with a supportive team and a positive community that cheers them on. Nothing makes you feel as good as oxytocin.

Community is also key for healing. I can't emphasize this enough. Isolation hurts us; community unites us. Lean in to the community of other women as you build this amazing healing lifestyle for yourself. Gather a few friends and fast together. Exercise together. Cheer each other on. Lift each other up. Fail a few times together. But enjoy the experience of trying a new approach to health. Have fun with it. Healing should be a community experience in which everyone wins.

LIFESTYLE CONSIDERATIONS

Most women discover that fasting becomes a way of life that they can sustain for years to come. With that in mind, I want to give you a few thoughts about how to best make this new lifestyle work for you.

Relationships

This consideration is at the top of my list. Here's why: There are many factors in your life that will determine how healthy you are, and your relationships are definitely one of them. Having good, positive, supportive relationships is key to living a healthy life. Not to forget the oxytocin burst you get from making sure you are surrounded by people you love. Let's make sure that as you learn the art of fasting you are still able to sit down and eat with the ones you love. Remember that a fasting lifestyle should be fun and flexible, allowing you to be in community with those you love while still thriving with your health.

One question I get often is how to fast around the demands of a family. The kids' lunches you make in the morning, the family dinner you sit down to at night, different food preferences . . . how do you build your fasting lifestyle around that? This is all customizable. You will see that fasting like a girl will allow you to meet these demands. Flexibility is at the root of a woman's fasting lifestyle.

Schedule

You will also see that varying your fasts and food allows you to match your fasting lifestyle to any circumstance. Perhaps the most challenging schedule I have had to create a fasting lifestyle for has been for actress Kat Graham. She reached out to me when shooting a movie that was being filmed at night. Talk about messing up your circadian rhythm! The nighttime schedule forced her to go to sleep at 6 A.M. and start her day at noon. With long days and an irregular schedule her energy was plummeting, so we needed to create a fasting lifestyle that powered up her mitochondria. At the time she was not fasting, so I taught her how to do short intermittent fasts, drinking coffee with some MCT oil in it until early evening and then breaking her fast with a protein-rich vegetarian meal, leading her right into her prime filming time. This small twist to her fasting lifestyle brought her energy back and helped her get through the rigors of that film shoot.

Activity level

Adapting your fasting lifestyle to meet your activity level can be key. Whether you are a high-performing athlete or just need more fuel for a long day at the office, you can adapt your fasting and eating windows according to what your energy output requires. I have seen high-performing women build fasting lifestyles around the times in which they need to be at their best. One of my patients, Susie, was a 37-year-old marathon runner. In a weekly routine, she had some runs that were lower in mileage, while other days she really stretched her runs, going long distances. We built her fasts and foods around her workout schedule while taking into consideration her hormonal fluctuations. Through a customized approach that had her leaning in to longer fasts on the lower-mileage days and shortening her fasting windows on the days leading up to her longer runs, Susie not only gained more stamina, she also improved her times. If you have high physical or mental demands on you, building a fasting lifestyle will enhance your performance, not deplete you.

Hopefully you are seeing a pattern here. You are unique, so varying your fasts and food to meet your hormones and lifestyle will improve your performance and the joy you experience in any endeavor of your life.

A great example of how you can take these fasting lifestyle pillars and transform your health is with Kathy, a member of my private fasting group, the Reset Academy. As a 45-year-old perimenopausal woman who struggled with type 2 diabetes and obesity, she was close to 100 pounds overweight and was on a collision course with poor health—and she knew it. She often found herself in her doctor's office searching for answers, only to leave frustrated by his lack of advice about lifestyle changes she could make. His only recommendations were to lose weight and watch her sugar intake. But how was she to go about that? She had tried weight-loss gimmicks for years only to regain the weight. She was ready to take action and desperately wanted a way out of her blood sugar dysregulation and dependency on medications.

Taking matters into her own hands, Kathy went to YouTube to better understand the underlying causes of type 2 diabetes. Now let's just stop and think about this for a moment. The fact that Kathy's doctor was ill-equipped to give better nutritional advice left her feeling disempowered and forced her to have to look for solutions elsewhere. The upside of social media is that you can teach yourself how to solve many of your health challenges. This is a huge paradigm shift that has been occurring in the world of health care. The advice many doctors and health experts give on these platforms can be solid. It just takes tenacity to find the right information for you. Well, Kathy found the right information in the world of fasting.

Her first step was to train herself to do intermittent fasting. Within a few months she dropped 20 pounds. She was so encouraged by the results that now she was open to evaluating her food choices. She paired her intermittent fasting lifestyle to the Whole30 diet, dropping even more weight. Each new pound that fell off motivated her. She was requiring less medication, her blood sugar numbers were going down, and for the first time in years she felt like she was in control of her health again.

After intermittent fasting for a few months, Kathy decided to play with her food choices more. She learned about the ketogenic diet and realized that lowering her carbohydrate load could accelerate her weight-loss results. By then fasting had become so helpful to her health efforts that she was eating only one meal a day. Pairing an extremely low-carbohydrate version of the ketogenic diet to her one-meal-a-day fasting lifestyle gave her insane results. Nine months after Kathy sat in the doctor's office that day looking for lifestyle solutions to her chronic health problems, she was 70 pounds lighter.

You are the miracle, not the diet. As we continue through this fasting journey together, always keep in mind that as a woman your hormones drive every aspect of your life. As much as we may not like it, our hormones are always in control. Whether you are 25 or 65, your hormonal surges are complex. This is why your fasting lifestyle will look vastly different from your husband's, brother's, son's, or male best friend's. Don't compare your fasting efforts to theirs. You can put a man on a fast and he often will get results quickly. It doesn't always happen that way for women. Stay positive and in your hormonal lane.

If you feel frustrated at any point on your fasting journey, I want to remind you that there is no such thing as failure when it comes to fasting. If you have a day when you feel like you've failed, remind yourself it's just feedback. Keep learning. Don't give up. It's in that frustration that you grow new neurons in your brain. Failure is necessary for long-term success. Building a fasting lifestyle will give you results like you've never seen before, but you will have moments of setbacks. Keep in mind that knowledge can fuel you, so go back and reread chapters if need be, but know that the only way you'll fail at a fasting lifestyle is by quitting. You've got this! I am here with you every step of the way.

CHAPTER 6

Foods That Support Your Hormones

Food is not our enemy. In fact, the right foods can ignite our incredible hormonal superpowers. It's our approach to food that has gone wrong. Just like we haven't been taught how to fast like a girl, most of us never got the memo that we need to eat differently at different times of our menstrual cycle. We let our taste buds choose the foods we eat, not our hormones. When you learn to eat with your hormones, you literally can have your cake and eat it too.

Much like building a house starts with a good foundation, eating to support your hormones starts with a strong foundation, built on four principles: ingredients matter, glycemic load, diversity, and cycling. Once you understand these principles, eating for your hormonal needs will become more intuitive.

FOOD PRINCIPLE #1-INGREDIENTS MATTER

When I was growing up, I would often go to the grocery store with my mother. And like any other kid, I always begged her to buy me a treat as we snaked through the aisles. So she started a game with me. Every time I saw something I wanted, I had to read her the first four ingredients. If sugar landed in those first items, I couldn't buy it. One time I really wanted Fruit Roll-Ups. All the kids at school had them in their lunches, and they would wrap them around their fingers and suck on them with such glee. I so desperately wanted in on the fun. And how bad could they be? After all they were called FRUIT Roll-Ups! But their number one ingredient was sugar, so it was a no-go. As frustrating as it was, my mom taught me an important lesson: Ingredients matter.

When you look at a food label, the top section is a chart that tells you the nutritional breakdown of the food, and the bottom part is the list of ingredients. Most of us have been conditioned to look at the top section and go straight to the calories. Unfortunately, counting calories does nothing for our hormonal health. The list of ingredients, on the other hand, greatly impacts your hormones. Train yourself to go to the ingredient list first. Good healthy ingredients like healthy oils, organic fruits and vegetables, and grass-fed proteins support great hormonal production, while fake, chemical-laden ingredients have been associated with altering your natural hormone production and contributing to metabolic disease.

As you look at that ingredient list, there are a couple of questions I encourage you to ask yourself. The first is, How long is the list? Typically, the longer the list of ingredients, the more possible chemicals have been put into that food. Think about when you are looking at a recipe for the first time. How many ingredients will it take to make that recipe? Five to eight maybe? Today's nutrition labels are not only extremely long but are packed with ingredients that are hard to understand. One easy rule to remember is if an ingredient list has more than five ingredients, put the item back on the shelf. The more ingredients, the more opportunities for a chemical or two to slip in.

The second question to ask yourself is whether you recognize the ingredients. The quality of food matters greatly. When you read an ingredient list, ask yourself whether you would know where to find that ingredient in your grocery store. If you have never heard of the ingredient and wouldn't know what grocery aisle it might be in, there is a good chance it's a synthetic ingredient that has the potential to destroy your health.

Toxic ingredients to avoid

A harsh truth is that gone are the days when all the ingredients in foods were safe. For many food companies, shelf life and profits have become more of a priority than your health, which is why we have seen an uptick in toxic ingredients in our foods. Some of these may look familiar to you. Pesticides, preservatives, dyes, and artificial flavors are all common food label ingredients. A good rule of thumb is if you can't pronounce it, chances are it's a chemical.

It can be hard to wrap your head around the fact that ingredients that could potentially harm our health are able to get into our foods in the first place. Shouldn't there be regulations around the health status of ingredients? Well, there used to be. Unfortunately, the rules around what is deemed safe in food products have changed dramatically over the past few decades. A new category has been created for emerging ingredients. It's called GRAS, or "generally recognized as safe." Ingredients that go into this category are considered safe until proven not to be. Instead of having to spend years and hundreds of thousands of dollars proving an ingredient's safety, food companies can expedite the approval by having it evaluated by a panel of experts from the Food and Drug Administration. If there is no clear evidence of harm, despite the lack of long-term research, the ingredient can be categorized as GRAS. In the past 20 years, more than 50,000 ingredients have fallen into the category.

An example of a common GRAS ingredient that was allowed in our foods and then later found to be harmful is partially hydrogenated oil. In 2015, after years on the GRAS list, partially hydrogenated oils were proven to cause cardiovascular disease, forcing food companies to pull them from their products.[1] Yet for 60 years partially hydrogenated oils went unchallenged. This lack of regulation by the FDA has many consumer protection groups concerned and is something you should be aware of. I encourage you to stay away from the foods that have ingredients in them that you don't recognize. The more mysterious an ingredient sounds, the more suspicious I would be of it. A few examples of GRAS list ingredients include sorbitol, sodium aluminum phosphate, BHA and BHT preservatives, nitrates, and nitrites.

To confuse matters even more, there are some ingredients that might sound benign but can be harmful—like natural flavorings. Isn't natural what we are going for with our food? Yes, but we need to look deeper into what *natural* means. The FDA defines a natural flavor as "a substance extracted, distilled, or similarly derived from plant or animal matter, either as is or after it has been roasted, heated, or fermented, and whose function is for flavor, not nutrition." The key part of that definition being that the purpose of this vague ingredient is flavor, not nutrition. There are an estimated 3,000 food additives that can be placed into the category of natural flavors. According to the Environmental Working Group, many of these flavorings are chemicals, carrier solvents, and preservatives such as propylene glycol, polyglycerol esters of fatty acids, mono- and diglycerides, benzoic acid, and polysorbate 80.[2] One of the natural flavoring ingredients you may know is actually monosodium glutamate, a proven neurotoxin that has been scientifically linked to obesity, neurodegenerative brain disorders like Alzheimer's, and reproductive abnormalities.[3]

As confusing as this all may sound, there are some simple questions you can ask yourself that will ensure you don't end up with a food that is packed with hormone-destroying chemicals.

- How long is the ingredient list?
- What are the first few ingredients?
- Do you recognize the ingredients?
- Do any of the ingredients sound like a chemistry experiment?
- What kind of oils, sugars, and flours are listed?
- Do you see any artificial colors, flavors, or dyes listed?

You want to look at that list and feel like the food you are about to eat is made in nature, not a chemistry lab. Bottom line: Nature's foods—those that come straight from the ground—are going to be best for your hormones. Take the potato versus a potato chip. A potato you buy from your store and cook at home is going to be more nutritious than a bag of potato chips that have been cooked in harmful oils and sprayed with toxic chemicals. A chemical that is commonly sprayed on potato chips is acrylamide, which has been shown to cause cancer in animal studies and nerve damage in factory workers who are exposed repeatedly.[4]

Foods to add

Once you start to recognize these ingredients and avoid them, then you can focus on what you can eat. Good-quality foods will support your health in many ways. You will notice that I said *foods*, not *ingredients*. The best-quality foods don't have an ingredient list. Fresh produce is an example. An apple doesn't require a label because it is in its original form, no alterations needed. Once you start altering or adding to the original food, you will see an ingredient list placed on that food. In general, a good rule to follow when you enter your grocery store is to stick to the perimeter of the store. This is where the fresh, chemical-free foods tend to live. Good-quality foods fall into three categories: They support your hormone production, they build your muscles, and they grow your gut microbiome.

Hormone-supporting foods

Your sex hormones—estrogen, progesterone, and testosterone—are greatly influenced by what you eat. If you were at a restaurant and these hormones were ordering for you, they would each request something different. Understanding what each of these hormones craves is key to using food to your hormonal advantage.

Estrogen thrives when you keep glucose and insulin low. If estrogen were doing the ordering, it would request a salad over a sandwich. Bread spikes your blood sugar, which is not to estrogen's liking. Once your period starts and your body ramps up your estrogen levels, leaning in to a low-carbohydrate diet through your ovulation can give estrogen a chance to shine. If you are a menopausal woman who is dealing with rapidly declining estrogen levels, a low-carb diet can feel like a life ring that gets thrown your way to save you from weight-loss resistance, mental fogginess, and hot flashes. Women struggling with fertility due to an absence of healthy estrogen can lean in to the ketogenic diet to bring back normal ovulation. There are so many reasons why I love the ketogenic diet, but for women I love it the most for its influence on regulating estrogen. Imbalances in estrogen are prevalent among too many women. Estrogen dominance is contributing to skyrocketing hormonal cancer rates, while estrogen depletion is sending menopausal women into a hormonal frenzy. At the root of both of these estrogen extremes lives insulin resistance. Yet too many women don't know they are insulin resistant.

Outside of keeping your carbohydrate load low, there are several foods that estrogen would love for you to add in. The first is good fats, specifically foods that are naturally high in cholesterol. Cholesterol is a precursor to making estrogen, and any food that supports healthy cholesterol production is a win for estrogen. If the thought of raising cholesterol levels scares you, remember there is good cholesterol and bad cholesterol. To make estrogen you need more of the good cholesterol known as high-density lipoprotein, or HDL. This healthy cholesterol is so crucial for estrogen that your miraculous body will change your cholesterol levels throughout your menstrual cycle, elevating your HDLs at the moments in your cycle that you need more estrogen.[5] How cool is that?! You can use your diet to your advantage to ensure that your body has enough healthy cholesterol to efficiently make estrogen.

Estrogen also loves healthy phytoestrogens, which are plant-based compounds that mimic estrogen. When these compounds enter your body, they bind to estrogen receptor sites and your body will treat them as if they are estrogen. The most popular phytoestrogen you may know is soy. Although soy has gotten a bad reputation for contributing to hormonal cancers like breast and ovarian, current research is proving that organic soy can help support the production of protective estrogen.[6] When it comes to food and estrogen, there is a lot of mixed messaging around foods that support healthy estrogen production and foods that cause the proliferation of toxic estrogens. Cycling small doses of organic soy into your diet in the form of tofu or edamame can support healthy estrogen production. But soy is not the only phytoestrogen powerhouse. Other phytoestrogens that are helpful and keep your blood sugar low include seeds and nuts, legumes, and fruits and vegetables.

FOODS THAT SUPPORT ESTROGEN

GOOD FATS

- Olive oil
- Flaxseed oil
- Sesame seed oil
- Avocados

SEEDS AND NUTS

- Brazil nuts
- Almonds
- Cashews
- Roasted salted peanuts
- Pine nuts
- Pumpkin seeds
- Sunflower seeds
- Walnuts
- Sesame seeds

LEGUMES

- Peas
- Chickpeas
- Soybeans
- Lima beans
- Carob
- Kidney beans

- Mung beans
- Pinto beans
- Black-eyed peas
- Lentils

FRUITS AND VEGETABLES

- Sprouts
- Cabbage
- Spinach
- Onion
- Garlic
- Zucchini
- Broccoli
- Cauliflower
- Strawberries
- Blueberries
- Cranberries

A litany of health benefits can be attributed to consuming these phytoestrogens, including a lowered risk of osteoporosis, heart disease, breast cancer, and menopausal symptoms. Healthy estrogen production is also key for normal ovulation to occur. Within your menstrual cycle you will need the most estrogen production during the days leading up to ovulation, so adding in good fats and plenty of phytoestrogens is essential.

Progesterone is another hormone that is highly influenced by your food choices. Think of progesterone and estrogen as sisters. They may come from the same family and look very similar, but their personalities are vastly different. This means when it comes to food and fasting, we want to treat them uniquely. Where estrogen likes your blood sugar to be low, progesterone would prefer that you keep your blood sugar a little higher. Because of this it's common the week before your period to crave carbohydrates. If you are monitoring your blood sugar on a regular basis, you may notice that your blood sugar naturally elevates the week before your period. This is a normal response from your body to ensure that you have all the right components to make progesterone. Foods that support progesterone production will naturally be higher on the glycemic index. Potatoes, for example, will cause a higher blood sugar spike that helps give progesterone the glucose burst it needs. Yet be mindful that mixed with harmful oil, potatoes can become inflammatory very quickly. So, sorry, ladies, no french fries.

FOODS THAT SUPPORT PROGESTERONE

ROOT VEGETABLES

- White potatoes
- Red potatoes
- Sweet potatoes
- Yams
- Beets
- Turnips
- Fennel
- Pumpkin
- Butternut squash
- Acorn squash

- Honeynut squash
- Spaghetti squash

CRUCIFEROUS VEGETABLES

- Brussels sprouts
- Cauliflower
- Broccoli

TROPICAL FRUITS

- Bananas
- Mangoes
- Papaya

CITRUS FRUITS

- Oranges
- Grapefruit
- Lemons
- Limes

SEEDS

- Sunflower
- Flax
- Sesame

LEGUMES

- Chickpeas
- Kidney beans
- Black beans

Muscle-building foods

Your muscle strength matters greatly to your overall health. Research shows that women who focus on building muscle throughout their lives not only stay metabolically healthy but can build stronger bones, have less depression, and live longer. Building muscle isn't just an activity you do in the gym; it requires eating foods packed with protein. Protein stimulates a cellular healing pathway called mTOR. When we fast, we stimulate the autophagy pathway. When we eat, we stimulate mTOR. They are two opposing cellular healing mechanisms. If you are looking for a lean muscular look with your body, know that fasting is the tool to lean you out, while eating protein will help you grow stronger. It's a beautiful combination.

But choosing the right protein for your body is easier said than done. Like many foods you encounter daily, there are good and bad versions. When it comes to protein, there are two things to consider: quality and quantity. Let's begin with quality. Protein comes in two forms—animal and plant based. Both types of protein have pros and cons. Knowing what protein source works best for your health goals is important.

The key molecules that make up protein-rich foods are amino acids, which are essential not only for building muscle but also for keeping your brain and immune system working at their best. Amino acid deficiency can result in decreased immunity, digestive problems, depression, fertility issues, and brain fog. Because of the positive impact amino acids can have on many aspects of your health, you want to become familiar with foods that are rich with amino acids.

There are in total 20 different amino acids, 9 of which are considered essential, which means your body can't make them on their own, so you have to get them from an outside source. Animal protein packs the greatest amino acid punch, giving you all nine essential amino acids, while plant proteins don't have that same amino acid power. There is no one plant that has all nine essential amino acids, so you need to be sure to eat a good variety of plant-based foods to complete the amino acid profile your body needs. Many vegetarians find it helpful to add in an amino acid supplement because it's too difficult to eat the variety of plants to ensure they are getting a complete array of all nine aminos.

For building muscle there are three specific amino acids to focus on: leucine, isoleucine, and valine. Leucine is the most important. Animal-based foods that are high in leucine include chicken, beef, pork, fish, milk, cheese, and eggs. Plant-based proteins that give you leucine are pumpkin seeds, navy beans, and tofu. If you are a vegetarian wanting to build muscle, be sure you are eating enough leucine-dense foods. If you find those choices limited, you may want to add in a good amino supplement.

MUSCLE-BUILDING FOODS

LEUCINE-, ISOLEUCINE-, AND VALINE-RICH FOODS

- Chicken
- Beef
- Pork
- Fish
- Milk
- Cheese
- Eggs
- Pumpkin seeds

- Navy beans
- Tofu

With both animal- and plant-based foods, you want to make sure you skip the endocrine-disrupting chemicals. With plant-based diets it's the pesticides that are sprayed on foods that can negatively impact your hormones, whereas with animal-based proteins it's the added antibiotics and growth hormones that you need to avoid. The best approach to getting clean, healthy foods is to always choose organic, non-GMO, and antibiotic- and hormone-free foods whenever possible.

The second principle of protein to focus on is quantity. Using protein to build muscle requires that you eat enough of it. It takes 30 grams of protein at one meal to trigger mTOR and build your muscles stronger.[7] The amount becomes increasingly important as you age. After 40 years old, the amino acid sensors in our muscles start to weaken. When you are younger you often think of muscle as necessary to look good in a swimsuit, but as you age muscle becomes more critically important for functionality. Regardless of your age, the more muscle you have, the stronger you will feel and the better you will be at metabolically switching.

Microbiome-building foods

There are 10 times more bacterial cells in your body than human cells. And 90 percent of all the bacteria that lives in our bodies exists in our gut. When you eat healthily, you power up the good bacteria that lives in the inner mucosal lining of your gut. With the proper fuel, these bacteria break down estrogen for excretion, make neurotransmitters for your brain, balance your immune system, and provide you with melatonin to help you sleep. When you eat ultra-processed foods packed with bad oils, sugars, and chemical-laden ingredients, you kill your helpful bacteria and create an environment where harmful bacteria thrive. This sets you up for a very deficient microbiome, leading to anxiety, high blood sugar, low melatonin production, and an inability to break down estrogen for excretion. If this sounds like you, there's no need to panic yet. If you feed these bacteria the right foods, you can bring their vibrancy back in as little as three days.

Bacteria thrive on three types of foods: probiotic, prebiotic, and polyphenol foods. Probiotic foods have live microbes in them that support neurotransmitter production, vitamin metabolism, proper immune function, and lower inflammation. Probiotic foods are often fermented, such as sauerkraut or yogurt. Prebiotic foods feed the helpful microbes in your gut, allowing them to multiply. Prebiotic foods tend to contain more fiber, making them an excellent fuel for your microbiome. Polyphenols are mostly found in plant-based foods and not only nourish your gut microbes but also act as antioxidants.

For simplicity, I refer to these as the three Ps. A diet high in the three Ps will help you grow the good microbes that are critical to your hormonal health. The hormone-building foods I mentioned above help in the production of hormones, whereas the three Ps support a healthy microbiome that helps break down those hormones, making them usable to your cells and supporting healthy excretion. The beautiful part of eating for your microbiome is that the options are plentiful.

Probiotic-rich foods

The first P you want to focus on are probiotic-rich foods. It is estimated that you have more than 4,000 different species of bacteria in your gut that are all hard at work to keep you healthy. Throughout your life you have most likely been on a few rounds of antibiotics, undergone periods of chronic stress, or perhaps spent a few years on the birth control pill. These moments in your life have killed the good microbes in your gut. Adding in probiotic-rich foods is the quickest way to replenish a depleted supply. Among the most powerful are fermented foods, whereby microbes have been used to break down the sugars, lowering their glycemic load and packing a probiotic punch. The process of fermentation allows for helpful bacteria to grow within a food—that often gives it a sour taste. As such this will help add in new strains of helpful bacteria for your gut. The benefits of fermented foods are broad. They can be easier to digest, give you more vitamins and minerals than regular vegetables, improve symptoms of anxiety and depression, and power up your immune system. Each food you ferment can provide different healing effects. For example, one of the vegetables in kimchi is fermented scallion, which is known to boost viral immunity.[8] Kefir is fermentation of dairy that provides you with trillions of helpful bacteria that lowers bad cholesterol, blood pressure, and provides you with a surplus of antioxidants. Just make sure you keep an eye out for sugary additions to these low-glycemic treats.[9]

Luckily, fermented foods have become quite popular, and you can find all kinds of fermented vegetables and dairy products at your local store. Fermented foods are also easy and safe to make in your own kitchen. In Chapter 11, I will introduce you to several recipes using fermented foods that are easy to make at home.

PROBIOTIC-RICH FERMENTED FOODS

- Sauerkraut
- Kimchi
- Pickles
- Yogurt
- Kefir dairy
- Kefir water
- Kombucha

Prebiotic-rich foods

This brings me to the second P, prebiotic-rich foods. Think of the good bacteria in your gut as your favorite pet who makes you feel happy and loved and always puts a smile on your face. What would happen if you didn't feed this pet? Unfortunately, he would eventually die, wouldn't he? Well, the bacteria in your gut are the same. They will perform some amazing feats for your health, but you must feed them. What they love most are prebiotic foods. Some of the prebiotic foods that support a healthy microbiome look much like hormone-building foods, making them especially beneficial for women. The following are some of the most powerful prebiotic foods you can eat.

PREBIOTIC FOODS

- Chicory root
- Dandelion root
- Konjac root
- Burdock root
- Onions
- Jerusalem artichoke
- Garlic
- Leeks
- Asparagus
- Red kidney beans
- Chickpeas
- Split peas
- Cashews
- Pistachios
- Hummus

Polyphenol foods

The last P to add into your diet are polyphenol foods. Packed with antioxidants, polyphenol plant-based foods create an environment in the gut that allows a plethora of diverse microbes to thrive. If prebiotic foods feed the good bacteria in your gut, polyphenol foods create a nurturing home for them to replicate. Here's a fun fact: Two of the most polyphenol-dense foods are red wine and dark chocolate. But before you rush off to Napa Valley and binge on an expensive cabernet, keep in mind that the quality of these polyphenol foods matters. Luckily, we are seeing a surge in popularity of natural, low-alcohol wines that are free of harmful chemicals, are higher in polyphenols, and will support a healthy microbiome better than the commercial red wine you find in every grocery store. You can easily navigate a wine menu or your local wine shop by looking for key words like *biodynamic*, *organic*, or *sustainable*. You also want to look for wine that is less than 13 percent alcohol. The lower the alcohol, the less sugar that red wine will have. You want to approach chocolate with the same level of detail as you do red wine. Quality matters. Dark chocolate that is greater than 70 percent cacao, with minimal sugar added, will provide your microbiome a richer polyphenol experience than an everyday chocolate candy bar that most likely has large amounts of sugar.

The research on polyphenols is impressive. Polyphenol-dense foods help regulate your blood pressure, improve circulation, reduce chronic inflammation, protect you against neurodegenerative diseases, and can lower your blood sugar levels.[10] Like many of the foods that fall under the three Ps, most polyphenol foods are plant based. One surprising category of polyphenols includes herbs and spices. Often thought of as merely flavor enhancers, spices serve a bigger purpose than just improving taste. Cloves, for example, are not only tasty, they have one of the highest polyphenol counts and are proven to support a healthy liver and to lower blood sugar.[11] This can be a helpful spice to add into your diet that will support your fasting efforts. The list of foods that have the hormone-healing power of polyphenols should not be overlooked.

POLYPHENOL FOODS

- Artichoke hearts
- Broccoli
- Brussels sprouts
- Cloves
- Saffron
- Oregano
- Rosemary
- Thyme
- Basil
- Cinnamon
- Cumin
- Curry
- Dark chocolate
- Olives
- Parsley
- Red wine
- Shallots

Whether you are incorporating foods that support your hormones, build muscle, or feed your microbiome, the key is being intentional about it. All too often we let our taste buds drive our food decisions. As you build your fasting lifestyle, you will notice that your taste buds will change and your appetite will decrease. The bad cravings or voracious appetite will cease. I have experienced this firsthand. For most of my life I battled sugar and carbohydrate cravings. I also was that person who was often "hangry." You didn't want to be around me if I didn't eat every couple of hours. Once I learned how to customize fasting to my hormonal needs, my hunger and cravings went away. I know that sounds too good to be true, yet as you learn to fast like a girl you, too, will find that you crave food less. But beware: This makes it even more important to eat intentionally to support hormone production, muscle growth, and powering up your microbiome.

FOOD PRINCIPLE #2-GLYCEMIC LOAD MATTERS

The vital signs that doctors evaluate every time you step in their office are grossly missing one measurement—blood sugar. If there is one tool that will help you understand the direction your health is heading, it's your blood sugar. Blood sugar that is out of normal range can indicate that metabolic disease is brewing. Cardiovascular conditions, high blood pressure, elevated cholesterol levels, increasing waist circumference, diabetes, and fatty liver disease could often be prevented if a woman had a better understanding of the trends of her blood sugar levels. Although there are many things that influence your blood sugar, the foods you eat have the greatest impact. Yet every food you eat will impact your blood sugar differently. Luckily there is a system for evaluating a food's impact on your blood sugar numbers. It's called the glycemic index. The glycemic index ranks foods on a number scale of 1 to 100. Foods closer to 100 will spike your blood sugar higher than foods that rank closer to 1. Refined carbohydrates like those in a piece of bread tend to score the highest on this index. A piece of whole-wheat bread has a glycemic index of 59. A food with a lot of fiber and fat, like an avocado, has a glycemic index of 15. The more you eat foods that are lower on this index, the less insulin requirements are needed from your pancreas. When you choose foods low on the glycemic index, you reduce both glucose and insulin, making your fasting lifestyle feel effortless.

Your blood sugar is not influenced by calories; it's influenced by the macronutrients of food. Understanding these macronutrients, or what are often referred to as macros, and how they make your blood sugar go up or down is key to thriving with your metabolic health. Choosing macros that keep your blood sugar from spiking high will help you switch over to the fat-burner energy system quicker. Once this switch is made you will notice your energy increases, your weight drops more quickly, and your mental clarity improves. This is such an important concept, since at the root of all chronic disease are foods that constantly elevate your blood sugar.

There are three major macronutrients to focus on: carbohydrates, proteins, and fats. Each one of these macros impacts your hormones differently and will spike your blood sugar in unique ways. Carbohydrates raise your blood sugar the highest, protein the second highest, and fat will help you maintain an even blood sugar level and may even lower it. In order to be metabolically flexible, balance hormones, and train your body to be a fat burner, you want to keep your blood sugar as stable as possible. Getting to understand these macros is important.

Carbohydrates

The simplest way to understand carbohydrates is that they're a measurement of the sugar, starch, and cellulose in a food. Carbohydrates come in two forms: simple and complex. Simple carbohydrates will spike your blood sugar quickly and possibly even raise your blood sugar well beyond levels that your body can effectively handle. When your body can't process a sudden surge of glucose coming in from your food, it will find other places to store that sugar. The first two places it stores sugar are your liver and fat cells. If you are like many people who have been eating a Western diet for decades, your body has most likely stored a lot of glucose in your liver and fat. If this overwhelms you, the good news is that fasting allows you to go after all that stored sugar. The key when it comes to your current diet is to make sure that when you eat carbohydrates you are eating fewer simple carbohydrates and more complex ones. Since complex carbohydrates have more fiber in them than simple carbohydrates, they cause less of a rise in your blood sugar, allowing your cells to slowly take the sugar in, leaving less for storage in your liver and fat.

The easiest way to know if a carbohydrate is simple or complex is to ask yourself, Was this food made by man or by nature? Nature-made food is complex, having more fiber, which slows the absorption of sugars into your bloodstream. Nature-made carbohydrates also meet the requirements laid out in principle #1, supporting your muscles, hormones, and microbiome. When timed properly with your cycle, nature-made carbohydrates are a wonderful tool to help you thrive with your health.

Simple carbohydrates, on the other hand, will lead you down a path toward obesity, poor immune function, and estrogen dominance. These foods are fairly easy to spot; the majority of them have a long shelf life and take up center aisles of your grocery stores. This is because most simple carbohydrates are laden with sugar and preservatives so that they can last longer on your pantry shelf. Unfortunately, they have no nutritional value and do nothing to support your health. The foods that fall into this category are cookies, crackers, cereals, chips, breads, pastas, and the majority of processed foods. Simple carbs are void of fiber and will raise your blood sugar easily. With a quick spike of blood sugar comes a massive release of insulin. With the sudden rise in glucose and insulin, your body will find creative places to store the excess. The more times you do this in a day, the more your body will store the extra glucose and insulin as fat. When you look at yourself in the mirror and villainize the extra weight you see, I encourage you to remember that all the extra fat you see was your body's way of saving your life. It had a choice to store it in organs or as fat, and it chose fat—a much better choice that has no doubt extended your life.

Carbohydrate measurement

As we move into understanding how to measure these macros, it's important to know that fasting like a girl requires you measure net carbohydrates, not total carbohydrates. Net carbs are the total carbohydrate load of a food minus the fiber. The fiber in foods is helpful because it slows the absorption of sugars into your bloodstream. A carbohydrate without fiber, much like we find in simple carbohydrates, raises your blood sugar quickly. When a carbohydrate has fiber in it, the glucose spike is much more gradual, giving your body time to properly assimilate that sugar into your cells. This is a large reason why I recommend you swap out man-made carbohydrates for nature's ones. Nature knew what it was doing when it created carbohydrates. When you start to understand how your body was designed, you will see that we are quite compatible with nature. Complex carbohydrates made with nature's wisdom will quickly be your go-to carbohydrate.

Protein

You read about the power of protein on muscle building, but it's also important to understand what this macronutrient does to your blood sugar—a helpful tool for a woman learning to fast.

Protein can have a very positive effect on your blood sugar in three ways. The first is that protein breaks down into glucose at a slower rate than a carbohydrate. This means that it won't quickly raise your blood sugar and cause a surge of insulin to be released from your pancreas. Next, protein can also slow down the absorption of carbohydrates. This is helpful when you are eating a meal that has both protein and complex carbs. When you combine a carbohydrate with a protein in the same meal, you may notice that the glucose response is much slower. A great example of this combination would be eating a steak with a potato. A potato by itself can elevate your blood sugar quickly, often leading you down a path toward insulin resistance and inflammation. Pair that potato with maybe a little butter, steak, and a salad, and now you have less of a glycemic spike.

Another plus: Protein will often kill your hunger. Protein takes longer to digest, sending a signal to the brain that you are still full. Many women discover that using a protein-rich snack to break a fast can satisfy hunger, provide a burst of mental clarity and energy, and make the transition from a fasted state into eating much smoother.

Because of its influence on your blood sugar, I highly recommend favoring protein over simple carbohydrates, especially if you are transitioning from a six-meal-a-day, high-carb, low-fat diet to fasting. Incorporating more protein into your diet can help give you the momentum you need to succeed.

I have one caveat: You want to make sure that you don't eat too much protein. In the ketobiotic diet that I discuss later in the chapter, I recommend 75 grams per day. Much more than this, and your blood sugar can spike too high, making it hard for you to get into ketosis. Years ago, I had a friend who was practicing the ketogenic diet for the first time. She decided to remove all refined carbohydrates from her diet for a month. Initially she was hungry, so she found protein to be a helpful go-to food to kill her cravings and hunger. After a few months she stopped losing weight, so she reached out to me to troubleshoot. When I had her calculate the amount of protein she was eating every day, it ranged between 150 and 200 grams of protein, which is WAY too much! If weight loss is your goal, keeping protein in a moderate range, like 75 grams per day, will help ensure that your blood sugar doesn't spike too high and cause an insulin surge. For my friend, the large amount of protein was keeping her blood sugar high, making it difficult for her to metabolically move from a sugar-burning over to a fat-burning state. Once we brought her protein down to 75 grams, metabolic switching became much easier, and weight came off.

Fat

Fat is no doubt the glycemic hero of the day. Not only will fat stabilize your blood sugar, but it will also kill your hunger. If you have been living with the understanding that fat will harm your health, I encourage you to open your mind and look at fat with new eyes. Fat is your friend, not your enemy. Here's the key to mastering your fat intake: Not all fat is created equal. In fact, if there is one nutritional concept that mixes people up more than any other, it's the delineation between good fat and bad fat. This is key: Good fats nourish your cells; bad fats inflame them. You want to embrace good fats and avoid bad fats at all costs.

The outside of your cells is nourished by good fat. This membrane determines which nutrients stay in the cell and which toxins need to be released. Bad fats inflame this membrane, blocking nutrients from getting in and toxins from getting out. Good fats repair this membrane, so this cellular regulation can work to your health advantage. Because of your cellular needs, healthy fats are making a comeback and the fat-free days are quickly disappearing. The nutritional world is starting to recognize the importance of this macronutrient. Once you open your eyes to the healing power of good fat, you'll find that food products filled with good fat are aplenty.

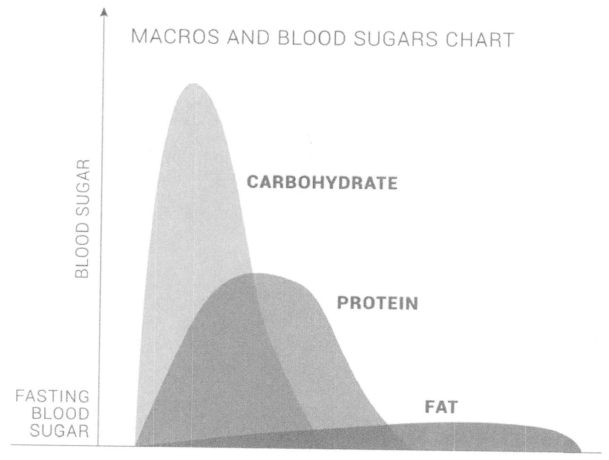

FOOD PRINCIPLE #3-DIVERSITY MATTERS

Diversity of food choices is one of the most overlooked nutritional ideas. As discussed above, different foods feed different gut bacteria. Limiting your food choices can restrict the growth of helpful microbes. When you stop and look at what you eat, I think you will find that you often eat the same things over and over. I know that the first time I looked at what I ate I was shocked at how I fell into a rut of eating the same foods repeatedly. If you want to help grow more healthy microbes, you are going to want to diversify your food choices.

The more variety you have in your food choices, the more your microbes can thrive. Different foods have different nutrients in them that feed different bacteria. Microbes are alive and have specific nutrient requirements to survive. For example, microbes within the *Prevotella* species grow best on carbohydrates. Dietary fiber provides a competitive advantage to bifidobacteria. And Bacteroidetes has a substrate preference for certain fats.[12] There are many stool tests that can help you determine which species you are low in, giving you a clear path toward which foods you may need to focus on to improve your microbial fitness.

Limiting the variety of your foods is often not a conscious choice. We can eat the same foods for a variety of reasons. Sometimes it's as simple as preference, convenience, or habit. If this idea of variation sounds like a daunting task, here's a good game to play. It's called the food diversity score. Look at the foods you eat and count all the different variations you consume in a week. Count everything from different vegetables and fruits to meats and even spices. The goal is to work to get up to 200 different types of food into your diet in one month. These foods should fall into one of these three categories: carbohydrates, protein, and fat. The carbohydrates that count are only complex carbs that come from nature. A simple carb like a cookie doesn't count. Spices do. This is where you can really diversify. Add different spices to your meals and your score will go up. This game helps keep me in check so that I am always on track with my diversity, keeping my gut happy. Some of my favorite spices to add into my diet to improve my plant diversity are:

- Cardamom
- Cumin
- Celery seed
- Onion powder
- Garlic powder

- Star anise
- Black pepper
- Turmeric
- Rosemary
- Thyme
- Basil
- Saffron
- Nutmeg
- Allspice
- Cloves
- Cinnamon
- Mustard seed

FOOD PRINCIPLE #4-CYCLING MATTERS

If diet variation feeds your microbes, cycling your food feeds your hormones. The beautiful part of being a woman is that we have a hormonal pattern that we can cycle our foods to, and I will teach you exactly that using the Fasting Cycle mapped out in Chapter 7. With estrogen coming in in the first part of our menstrual cycle, we can go ketobiotic and thrive, and then once we hit the week before our period, progesterone wants more complex carbohydrates, so we can switch to hormone feasting foods. If you are a postmenopausal woman or don't have a regular cycle, you can use the 30-Day Fasting Reset I lay out for you in Part III of this book to ensure that in a 30-day period you are properly cycling your food and fasts. Our hormones cycle, and so should our food and fasts. We can use our hormones as a guiding star to tell us exactly how to do that.

I realize that cycling adds another level of complexity to your food choices. The beauty of being a woman is that there is nothing simple about your body. Remember, your hormones are your superpowers and when you cycle your food choices with your hormonal surges, you will magnify these powers. In Chapters 8 and 9, I have laid out two ways for you to effortlessly know the best foods and fasts you can cycle to support your hormones. Once you understand your hormonal patterns, you will see that cycling your food to match those patterns is fun, easy, and will make you feel limitless.

PUTTING IT ALL TOGETHER

Now that you understand the four food principles, let's put them into a system that is easy to follow. There are two main styles of eating that work best for your hormones. One eating style will help regulate your blood sugar, allowing estrogen to flourish, while the other purposefully raises your glucose levels to support the needs of progesterone. These two styles of eating encompass all four food principles and give you a structure to follow throughout your menstrual cycle. If you don't have a cycle or are a postmenopausal woman, these styles are still helpful; you just won't track them to your cycle. In Chapter 8, I give you a 30-Day Fasting Reset to follow that will allow you to get the best of these food styles without timing them to an exact cycle.

KETOBIOTIC

Just like women need to fast differently, women need to do keto differently. Where a man can remove all carbohydrates and thrive on keto, women need more carbs and protein to make their sex hormones. When the ketogenic diet first became popular, I had some concerns. If you keep carbs to a minimum, where will you fit in vegetables and fruits? Nature has provided us with some incredible plant-based foods that dramatically support our health. Yet low-carb living can do wonders for your blood sugar, ability to burn fat, and improve healthy estrogen production. In an attempt to bring all of these great food concepts together, I created a version of the ketogenic diet called ketobiotic. The macros of this version of keto are slightly different from a traditional ketogenic diet. The "biotic" part of ketobiotic is critically important not only to enhance your microbial fitness but to get in the necessary food to feed the microbes that help you break down estrogen for detoxification.

Here's the simplest way to understand ketobiotic eating: You eat protein, a variety of vegetables and fruits, and load up on good fat. The rules for ketobiotic eating are as follows:

- Consume no more than 50 grams of net carbohydrates per day.
- Focus on natural carbohydrates such as vegetables and greens.
- Consume no more than 75 grams of clean protein per day.
- Greater than 60 percent of your food should be coming from good fat.

The benefits of ketobiotic eating are plenty. First, if you are looking to lose weight, the ketobiotic diet keeps glucose low, letting you switch into your fat-burning energy system much quicker. This also supports optimal estrogen production. Ketobiotic also takes into account a woman's need for more vegetables. Both your liver and gut thrive on vegetables. These two organs are essential for detoxification of harmful estrogens, so you want to make sure you are supporting them nutritionally.

Another reason this style works so well for women is the surge of ketones it triggers. Ketones heal, especially the master hormonal control center of your brain, hypothalamus, and pituitary. Ketobiotic provides you a beautiful combination of keeping glucose low, supporting your liver and gut, and using ketones to fuel your brain.

Hormone feasting foods

One of the challenges that many women faced when the ketogenic diet became popular is that they stopped eating foods that supported progesterone production. Hormone feasting foods bring these key nutrients back into your diet, boosting progesterone to elevate your moods, giving you better mental cognition, and helping you sleep better at night.

Hormone feasting foods are higher in carbohydrates. This purposely provides you with more nutritional support to produce progesterone. Hormone feasting days are going to increase your blood glucose levels and most likely will kick you out of ketosis. This is intentional. This is important for progesterone production. Hormone feasting also allows you to eat more fruits, including berries, apples, citrus, and tropical fruits, giving your gut microbes new fuel that it does not get on your ketobiotic days.

The rules for hormone feasting days are as follows:

- Consume no more than 150 grams of net carbs per day.

- Focus on nature's carbohydrates such as root vegetables and fruits.

- Consume no more than 50 grams of protein per day.

- Consume healthy fats as desired.

I discovered hormone-building days in my late 40s, when my progesterone levels were plummeting faster than what was age appropriate. Keto and long days of fasting were working so well for my weight and mental clarity that I kept my carbohydrate load too low all month long. This was contributing to erratic cycles, thinning hair, and surges of anxiety. I needed to find a food fix to maximize my progesterone production. As much as I love using fasting as a tool for healing, when it comes to building up progesterone, food is the tool. And the foods that build progesterone are incredibly yummy to eat—foods like squashes, beans, quinoa, potatoes, grass-fed beef, and tropical and citrus fruits. (I have a more complete list of some of my favorite hormone feasting foods in Appendix B.) Varying in hormone feasting days at the right moment of my cycle was magic for my progesterone production and quickly resolved my unwanted symptoms.

The biggest mental hurdle I see many women face with hormone-building days is their concern about gaining weight. A huge concept I want you to grasp is that when you eat and fast to meet your hormonal needs, weight will drop off even though at times you may feel you are eating a lot more carbohydrates. I know that sounds crazy, but that is a major benefit to a fasting lifestyle. It's when we live in opposition to our hormones that weight tends to stick around. Both ketobiotic and hormone feasting are styles of eating that promote health. Extra weight can be a sign of poor health. Trust as you learn to fast and eat in rhythm with your hormones that the weight will naturally disappear.

The easiest way to approach these two styles of eating is that when hormones are peaking at ovulation and a week before your period, you want to feed them, so you move into hormone feasting foods. When your hormones are at their lowest levels, during the first 10 days of your cycle and the 5 days post ovulation, you want to go into ketobiotic to keep insulin low. The switch between these two styles of eating lets you mimic the feast/famine cycling your primal ancestors thrived on, all timed perfectly to your hormonal needs.

Ready to put all of this information together in a usable plan that's right for you? In the next chapter, you are going to learn a tool called the Fasting Cycle. This tool unifies all the concepts you've learned up until now and gives you a strategy to time your fasts and food to your menstrual cycle.

CHAPTER 7

The Fasting Cycle

A woman's body is complex, so fasting is much different from just avoiding food for 13 hours. Unlike men, we have all sorts of hormones to think of, so timing our fasts to our menstrual cycle is critical. But the results are amazing: When timed properly, you will balance your hormones, supercharge your energy, turn into an incredible fat burner, and stave off disease. There is a lot to juggle here, but I created a concept called the Fasting Cycle to simplify it for you. I want you to think of the Fasting Cycle as a map. As with all maps, you can choose several different routes to get to the same destination. You have options. The Fasting Cycle gives you that same flexibility with the six fasts I laid out in Chapter 2. Once you understand the key concepts behind the Fasting Cycle, you'll see in the next chapter how we put it into action in the 30-Day Fasting Reset.

HOW THE FASTING CYCLE WORKS

First and foremost, the Fasting Cycle breaks down your menstrual cycle into three phases: the Power Phase, the Manifestation Phase, and the Nurture Phase, all named for the hormones influencing your moods in each phase. These names are designed to help you remember what the focus of each phase is. For example, during the power phase, your focus can be to lean in to longer fasts to accelerate healing, whereas during the nurture phase, you want to slow down with your fasting efforts and nurture yourself more with healthy foods.

Although the Fasting Cycle is built around a 30-day period, every woman has a different-length cycle. If your cycle is 28 days, then you will use this fasting system up to the 28th day. Once your period starts, you move to day one again. If you have a 32-day cycle, keep following the guidelines of the last phase—your nurture phase—until your period starts, then start the cycle anew.

There is no one-size-fits-all approach here. While I give you fasting and food suggestions for each cycle, experiment with each option and see what works best for you. Using the 30-Day Fasting Reset as a starting plan to encompass this fasting philosophy will help. If you are new to fasting, don't have a regular cycle, or are postmenopausal, the 30-Day Fasting Reset outlined in the next chapter will give you more structure to put this fasting philosophy into action. Once you understand what fasting like a girl feels like, you can experiment with longer fasts using the Fasting Cycle as your guide.

Remember, stretching your fasts out a little longer than you may be used to creates a hormetic response in your cells. As you have learned, lovingly encouraging our bodies to adapt to new stressors is a beautiful way to accelerate the healing process. Don't be shy to try some of the longer fasts; just make sure to do them at the right phase of your cycle.

There is a tremendous amount of healing that can happen as you find your fasting rhythm. Take one of my patients, where I had her try the Fasting Cycle system to help her overcome infertility. At 35 years old, Amy wanted so desperately to get pregnant. Her ob-gyn told her that it would be nearly impossible for her to conceive a baby until she lost weight. She had been obese for many years and tried every diet in the book with very little success. She had given up thinking that any diet would work for her. She and her husband tried to get pregnant for years and were close to pulling the trigger on expensive IVF treatment. Disheartened by her doctor's recommendations that her only path to pregnancy was through weight loss, Amy knew she had to try a different approach. Somewhere along her research on fertility, she found fasting. Could fasting be the tool she was missing for weight loss and fertility? Not realizing the importance of timing her fasts with her cycle, she started learning the strategies to fasting and got results quickly. Weight started to fall off her for the first time in her life. She was so pleased with her fasting experience, with the exception of one result: She lost her cycle. Although she was happy with her weight, not having a cycle was a massive problem for a woman who wanted to get pregnant.

More discouraged than ever, she took the advice of a friend, who turned her on to my YouTube channel. Amy devoured all the videos I've done on fasting for women. She had hoped that timing her fasts to her hormones would give her the weight-loss results she craved while still allowing her to get pregnant. Desiring the quickest result possible, Amy joined my Reset Academy and started asking questions on our weekly calls. I taught her how to customize her fasting lengths, using the Fasting Cycle to help regulate her hormones and bring back her periods. Once she found a fasting rhythm that matched to her menstrual cycle, her periods were back, and her weight was the best it had been in years. Four months after doing this new fasting regime, Amy was pregnant. I am not joking when I say fasting can be your hormones' best friend or worst enemy—it all depends on how you vary it.

HOW TO USE THE FASTING CYCLE

Three phases, five hormones, six different fasting lengths, two core eating styles: Are you ready to learn how to use this tool? Let's dive into each phase so that you can get to know them better.

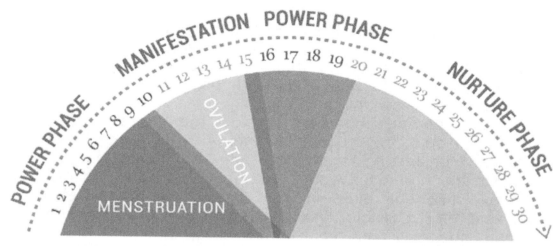

THE POWER OF FASTING AND YOUR CYCLE

DAY 1-10	DAY 11-15	DAY 16-19	DAY 20-BLEED
POWER PHASE	MANIFESTATION	POWER PHASE	NURTURE PHASE
(MENSTRUATION)*	(OVULATION)*		
FASTING:	FASTING:	FASTING:	NO FASTING
13-72 HOURS	13-15 HOURS	13-72 HOURS	
FOOD:	FOOD:	FOOD:	FOOD:
KETOBIOTIC	HORMONE FEASTING	KETOBIOTIC	HORMONE FEASTING

FASTING CYCLE

The Power Phases (Days 1–10 and 16–19)

Suggested fasting lengths: 13–72 hours
Optional food style: ketobiotic
Hormone focus: insulin, estrogen
Healing focus: autophagy and ketosis

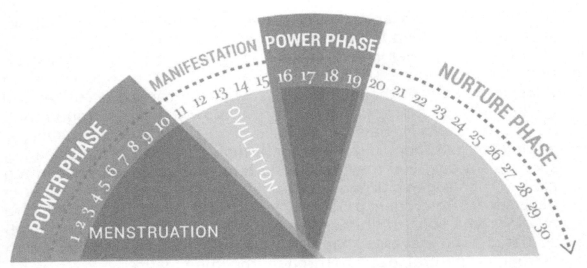

THE POWER OF FASTING AND YOUR CYCLE

DAY 1-10	DAY 11-15	DAY 16-19	DAY 20-BLEED
POWER PHASE (MENSTRUATION)•	MANIFESTATION (OVULATION)•	POWER PHASE	NURTURE PHASE
FASTING:	FASTING:	FASTING:	NO FASTING
13-72 HOURS	13-15 HOURS	13-72 HOURS	
FOOD:	FOOD:	FOOD:	FOOD:
KETOBIOTIC	HORMONE FEASTING	KETOBIOTIC	HORMONE FEASTING

POWER PHASE

There are times in your cycle when aggressive fasting (longer than 17 hours) is welcomed and times when it is not. Your power phases are those when you can maximize all the healing fasting can muster up, largely because this is the time when your sex hormones are at their lowest levels. During your menstrual cycle you have two such low points: one when you first start bleeding and the second one after you ovulate. It is often during these days that you feel more emotionally stable, have more energy, and are less hungry, making it a great time to fast longer.

In the first power phase (days 1–10), your body is focused on producing estrogen. You need estrogen to signal to your ovaries to release an egg. Without estrogen, ovulation cannot occur. At the beginning of this phase, your body will slowly make estrogen, and as you get closer to day 10 of your cycle, your body makes a larger amount of estrogen. If you are on a high-carbohydrate diet eating six meals a day, you may be inadvertently keeping your insulin too high for estrogen's liking. Excessive insulin not only creates a deficiency in estrogen production, but long term it can lead to a hyper-production of testosterone. This is your classic PCOS scenario. The reverse happens for menopausal women. With estrogen's natural decline through the menopause years, insulin resistance becomes more prevalent. It's a seesaw. When insulin goes up, estrogen goes down, and vice versa.

The second power phase (days 16–19) has another large dip in your hormonal production. At this point in your cycle, you are coming off the hormonal surges that happen in the manifestation phase. You might feel a downward shift in your libido and less mental clarity, motivation, and energy. Because your hormone levels are at a lower point, this small four-day window is another great opportunity to go into some of the fasts that are longer than 17 hours to stimulate autophagy, repair your gut, burn more fat, improve dopamine pathways, or reset your immune system.

The two healing processes you want to trigger here are autophagy and ketosis. While the shorter fasts (less than 17 hours) improve your fat-burning capabilities, longer fasts are where you'll see lasting repair of your cells happen. Certain areas of your body are more responsive to autophagy than others. The neurons that make up the hormonal control centers of your brain and the outer thecal cells of your ovaries repair incredibly well with autophagy. This is great news for your hormones. Healthy and balanced hormonal production requires your brain and ovaries to be healthy. Years of high insulin and repetitive toxic exposure can cause these two body parts to become sluggish, putting your hormones on a wild ride. Much like your sink can get backed up if it's clogged with waste, toxins and high insulin clog the cells in your brain and on your ovaries, challenging hormonal production as a result. Periodically stimulating autophagy will quickly repair this system. Just make sure you do it during your power phases.

If autophagy cleans your cells, the state of ketosis provides ketone fuel to power your cells up. Ketones are like rocket fuel for your mitochondria. Much like you need to charge your cell phone to keep it running, your mitochondria need a periodic ketone charge to keep them performing at their best. Autophagy and ketosis during your power phases provide a wicked healing combination for the organs that manage your hormones. This makes it a great time to go into longer fasts to ensure that these organs are juiced up and ready for the next phase of hormone production.

As far as the best food choices for your power phases, I highly recommend keeping glucose and insulin low. This makes the ketobiotic way of eating ideal at this time. Lowering your intake of carbohydrates while raising your intake of good fats and keeping protein in moderation is the perfect style of eating to pair with your fasts. In my power phases I often fast for 17 hours, break my fasts with good fats like an avocado with sauerkraut drizzled with flaxseed oil, and then for dinner I'll have a grass-fed steak and a large salad. I save my fruit and starches like sweet potatoes for my hormone feasting days. You will find some great ketobiotic recipes in Chapter 11 and a list of favorite ketobiotic foods in Appendix B.

The Manifestation Phase (Days 11–15)

Suggested fasting length: <15 hours
Optional eating style: hormone feasting foods
Hormone focus: estrogen, testosterone
Healing focus: supporting a healthy gut and liver

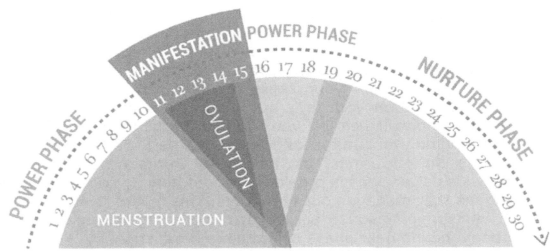

THE POWER OF FASTING AND YOUR CYCLE

DAY 1-10	DAY 11-15	DAY 16-19	DAY 20-BLEED
POWER PHASE	MANIFESTATION	POWER PHASE	NURTURE PHASE
(MENSTRUATION)•	(OVULATION)•		
FASTING:	FASTING:	FASTING:	NO FASTING
13-72 HOURS	13-15 HOURS	13-72 HOURS	
FOOD:	FOOD:	FOOD:	FOOD:
KETOBIOTIC	HORMONE FEASTING	KETOBIOTIC	HORMONE FEASTING

MANIFESTATION

If I had a favorite part of the monthly cycle, it would be the manifestation phase, when estrogen and testosterone peak and you get a mild surge of progesterone. All of these hormones line up in perfect synergy to help you feel your best. During this short five-day period, not only are you ready to make a baby, but the estrogen spike will spark creativity, beautify your hair and skin, and make you a great conversationalist. You also are an incredible multitasker when estrogen is high. But your hormonal bliss during this phase doesn't end with a huge surge in estrogen; you also get large amounts of testosterone at this time. This not only fires up your libido but also gives you a boost of motivation. If you want to run a marathon, time race day to this phase and you may surprise yourself with just how strong and powerful you feel. Is there a difficult conversation you need to have with someone? Time it for when your hormones are surging through you and enhancing your communication skills. Finally, during this time you get a small surge of progesterone, which gives you peace and calm. You truly were hormonally designed to feel incredible during this phase.

In the manifestation phase, we want to turn our healing focus from producing hormones to metabolizing them. Metabolizing a hormone means two things: breaking that hormone down into a usable form so it will be more readily used by your cells, and preparing that hormone for excretion. The two organs that help you metabolize hormones are your liver and gut. When these two organs are working at their best, your hormonal superpowers will peak during this time.

One hormone that is incredibly important to detoxify is estrogen. When estrogen is not broken down and excreted from your body, it stays stuck in your tissues. Unmetabolized estrogen leads to many hormonal cancers, including breast cancer, and contributes to a whole host of premenstrual symptoms such as breast tenderness, night sweats, moodiness, and even weight gain. Because of this you want to use the manifestation phase to support the breakdown and excretion of estrogen.

The best way to do this is to shift your focus from longer fasts as your healing tool to leaning in to foods that nourish your liver and gut. Hormone feasting foods will improve bile production for the breakdown of fats, improve digestion by stimulating the proper production of stomach acid and pancreatic enzymes, and support your body's absorption of key vitamins like B_{12} and iron.

The list of hormone feasting foods is long, but some of the ones that are especially important to support healthy hormone metabolism include:

- Cruciferous vegetables such as broccoli, brussels sprouts, and cauliflower

- Green leafy vegetables such as arugula, frisée, kale, and watercress
- Bitter lettuces such as radicchio, nettles, endive, and dandelion leaves
- Sesame and flaxseeds
- Fermented foods such as sauerkraut, kimchi, and yogurt
- Salmon
- Blueberries, raspberries, and boysenberries
- Apple varieties such as green and Newtown Pippins
- Green and dandelion teas
- Spices such as turmeric, cumin, saffron, and dill

When it comes to fasting during this phase, it's important to keep your fasts under 15 hours. Remember the reasons why women need to fast differently? One reason is because hormone surges can release toxins that have been stored in your tissues. If you are in a fasting state longer than 17 hours triggering autophagy, you may create more of a detox reaction, like nausea, vomiting, brain fog, lethargy, anxiety, or muscle aches. This can make for a really uncomfortable manifestation period. It's a time when you should be thriving, but you can feel horrible if you don't shorten your fasts and lean in to hormone feasting foods.

Now what about testosterone? It is in the manifestation phase that you are supposed to get your largest testosterone surge. Testosterone is a wonderful hormone for women. It gives us motivation and drive, plus it fires up our libido. If you are not feeling these traits at this time, you could be low in testosterone. Food and fasting is not your best tool for improving testosterone production. Removing toxins and major stressors from your life are the most impactful steps you can take to balance your testosterone levels. Phthalates are highly destructive to your testosterone production; these toxins act like a synthetic version of testosterone, which enables them to enter your cells. Much like a synthetic version of estrogen is not usable to your cells, synthetic testosterone is also useless. Unfortunately, phthalates are most commonly found in plastics, and personal care products with strong fragrances like those found in commercial perfumes, shampoos, and lotions. Although avoiding phthalates is a smart move for overall hormonal health, it will impact your testosterone levels the most. If you have signs of low testosterone, I strongly encourage you to avoid plastics and find natural sources for your beauty products and fragrances.

Stress can also come into play during this phase by suppressing the production of progesterone and testosterone, both of which require ample amounts of the steroid DHEA. Cortisol also needs DHEA in order to be produced. In a stressed state, your body will prioritize cortisol production over progesterone and testosterone. This can deplete your DHEA stores and leave you with low levels of these two sex hormones. In your manifestation phase, this might feel like loss of libido and motivation, and high states of anxiety—never a great combination. You can easily have your DHEA levels checked with a hormone test so you know for certain whether your stress levels are impacting these necessary hormones.

The Nurture Phase (Day 20–First day of your period)

Suggested fasting length: no fasting
Optional eating style: hormone feasting foods
Hormone focus: cortisol, progesterone
Healing focus: reducing cortisol

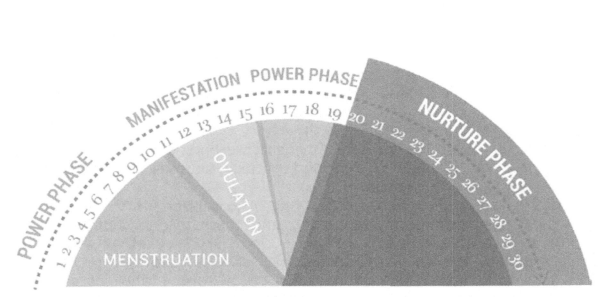

THE POWER OF FASTING AND YOUR CYCLE

DAY 1-10	DAY 11-15	DAY 16-19	DAY 20-BLEED
POWER PHASE	MANIFESTATION	POWER PHASE	NURTURE PHASE
(MENSTRUATION)•	(OVULATION)•		
FASTING:	FASTING:	FASTING:	NO FASTING
13-72 HOURS	13-15 HOURS	13-72 HOURS	
FOOD:	FOOD:	FOOD:	FOOD:
KETOBIOTIC	HORMONE FEASTING	KETOBIOTIC	HORMONE FEASTING

NURTURE PHASE

This is the phase of your cycle when you get to focus on you. Seriously! As women we so often give to others, leaving our own needs to be met last. Believe it or not, this has a hormonal consequence for us. Rushing around, constantly putting others' needs ahead of our own, and stressing our bodies with lack of sleep destroys one of the most important hormones we have: progesterone. Progesterone calms you and tells you everything is going to be okay. When we don't honor it during this week, we can feel like the world around us is spinning out of control. Hence the name of this phase: nurture. Take this week to nurture your body and watch progesterone shine.

There are three ways you can nurture yourself in this phase. The first is to skip fasting. The reason for this is that much like exercise, fasting can create small spikes in cortisol. Any increase in cortisol threatens the production of progesterone. Cortisol is also raised during excessive exercise. Pushing your body to extreme physical limits the week before your period can lead to depleted progesterone stores, so shift your workouts from higher-intensity activities to more nurturing activities like yoga, hiking, or long walks.

Your best food options during this nurture phase are back to hormone feasting foods. You can continue eating the foods you ate for liver and gut health during your manifestation phase, plus add in more starchy foods like potatoes, beans, and squashes (comfort food!). We are so brilliantly designed that our bodies are more insulin resistant during our nurture phase. This is for a good hormonal reason. Your body needs more glucose to make progesterone. Trying to get into ketosis during this time will be not only challenging for you but also destructive to progesterone. I have seen this all too often with women fasters and keto lovers. They feel so good with fasting and low-carb living that they want to keep going throughout their menstrual cycle. But your body was not designed to be in ketosis the week before your period. You may notice that your body craves more carbohydrates during this week. That is by design. It's a signal that you need to bring glucose back up. As glucose rises, progesterone will elevate, giving you a feeling of calm and preparing the uterine wall to shed. Once progesterone hits its peak, your period will start, and the fasting cycle starts all over again with your first power phase.

Raising glucose during this time isn't an excuse to dive into a tub of ice cream or box of pizza. You want to be strategic about the carbohydrates you eat during this phase. My favorite progesterone-building foods during the nurture phase are:

- Potatoes such as red, russet, Yukon Gold, purple, and new

- Sweet potato and yam varieties such as garnet and purple

- Squashes such as acorn, spaghetti, honeynut, and butternut
- Lentils and black beans
- Citrus fruits such as lemons, limes, grapefruit, and oranges
- Tropical fruits such as bananas, mangoes, and papaya
- Blueberries, raspberries, and boysenberries
- Pumpkin seeds
- Wild and brown rice and quinoa

I didn't fully understand how progesterone worked until I hit my perimenopausal years. As an overscheduled, type A woman I was constantly rushing, struggling to manage my stress, and fasting long hours. Nothing kills progesterone more than the rushing woman's lifestyle. Remember, your body doesn't know the difference between too much to do at work and being chased by a tiger (a leftover trait from prehistoric days). In order to run from that tiger, your body needs to take all of its hormonal resources and make cortisol so that you can sprint and get away. But the more you call on cortisol to get you through your day during this phase, the fewer resources you have for making progesterone. And without progesterone, your PMS symptoms will be at their worst, you will skip periods, and your uterus will be unable to hold a fertile egg. The name of the game during this phase is no tigers.

THE FASTING CYCLE AS A LIFESTYLE

Wherever you are on your fasting journey, I hope you find this cycle helpful. If you have been fasting for a while, I hope you see this fasting philosophy has been missing to help you time your fasts appropriately. I will keep encouraging you to experiment with the longer fasts. There is a world of healing that happens there. Just make sure that you use the Fasting Cycle to lean in to the longer fasts at the right hormonal time.

Now that you understand the fasting like a girl philosophy, let me give you a proven plan. The 30-Day Fasting Reset is a step-by-step plan that lets you vary your fasting lengths paired with the right food choices, all mapped to your menstrual cycle. If you don't have a cycle, no worries: This 30-day reset will be perfect for you to maximize your hormones regardless of what time of life you are in.

I'm not going to lie, fasting can get addictive. That might shock you right now, but after watching hundreds of thousands of women build fasting lifestyles, I will tell you that the moment you experience the results of fasting firsthand, you will want to move into longer and longer fasts. You've got this!

Never forget, your body is designed to self-heal. It has so many miraculous ways it repairs and resets you every day. When your health feels like a struggle, come back to the Fasting Cycle and ask yourself, "Am I living a life that is working with my hormones or against them?"

Ready to put all this information into action? Let's get you on your fasting journey.

PART III

THE 30-DAY FASTING RESET

CHAPTER 8

The 30-Day Fasting Reset

Welcome to your 30-Day Fasting Reset. I designed this reset to give you a clear plan that is founded on the philosophy of the Fasting Cycle. No need to reinvent the wheel. This reset will help you integrate the Fasting Cycle concepts into your life much quicker. Consider it a proven path where you know success will be the end result.

The 30-Day Fasting Reset has three essential criteria: First, it must metabolically flex you in and out of different-length fasts to provide enough of a hormetic stress so that your body adapts positively. Second, if you have a cycle, it needs to be timed to where you are in your cycle. If you don't have a cycle, it needs to supply all the neurochemical needs your hormones have in order to thrive. Lastly, resets are best done with a community.

METABOLICALLY FLEXING TO SATISFY ALL OF YOUR HORMONES

Although there are six different fasts that create a healing effect, for this reset you will use only three of those fasts. I purposely left the longest fasts out so that this 30-day reset would be approachable for most. If you have been fasting for a while and want a more challenging reset, I have mapped out an advanced version for you to try that encompasses a longer, 24-hour fast.

The three different-length fasts you will lean in to with this 30-day reset range from 13 hours to 20 hours. If you haven't fasted before, please make sure you do the two-week pre-reset work laid out below. This will make your 30-day reset experience much smoother. I will tell you this: During this 30-day reset you will have some uncomfortable moments. We actually welcome these moments because this is where healing happens. The principle of hormesis works only if enough stress is applied. If I were your personal trainer and every workout I gave you was easy and didn't push you, how quickly would you see results? Probably not very quickly. Creating intermittent moments that push you beyond your comfort zone will accelerate your healing. As you now know, your body was primally designed for it, so the moments of discomfort will come and go quickly.

In order to best prepare for those moments, I want you to think through what you will do when obstacles arise. One of the biggest reasons people fail at hitting their goals is because they don't plan for the obstacles that will inevitably show up. Whenever you are applying a hormetic stress to your fasting lifestyle, obstacles will appear. Some of the most common are hunger, boredom, detox symptoms, and lack of support. So acknowledge that possibility—it will make it much easier to navigate them when they do come your way. In Chapter 10, I will give you what I have seen work best for these obstacles so that you can ride them out smoothly.

TIMING YOUR FASTS TO YOUR CYCLE

This reset will take you through all the phases you learned with the Fasting Cycle. You will be moving in between no fasting, intermittent fasting, autophagy fasting, and a gut-reset fast. All are perfectly timed to your cycle. Now here is the hard part about creating a reset for women: All of you are in different places in your cycle. And some of you don't have a cycle.

If you do have a cycle, the first thing I want you to do if you are not already doing it is track your cycle. You want to start this reset on day one of your cycle and follow it all the way through until the moment you start to bleed again. If you have a 28-day cycle, then this will be a 28-day reset.

If you don't have a cycle, you can start this reset anytime you want and go all the way through for 30 days. This works fabulously for younger women who have lost their period and want it back, as well as for postmenopausal women who want to balance the hormones that might have gone on a wild ride throughout the menopause years. The beauty of this reset is that it has the power to pull you out of any imbalance you may have and get your hormones back in sync. Within a couple of months of repeating this reset all the way through, I consistently noticed that many mysterious hormonal problems cleared up without having to use any other mainstream therapies, like medications or supplementation. Many times within the first month of this reset, a woman in her reproductive years will start cycling again. For postmenopausal women, a month or two of this reset is the hormonal solution for lingering hot flashes, sleepless nights, and stubborn weight gain.

Postmenopausal Symptoms Alleviated with Fasting

- Lingering hot flashes
- Sleepless nights
- Stubborn weight gain
- Belly fat
- Mood changes such as depression and anxiety

RESETS DONE IN A COMMUNITY

Personally, I feel that all health endeavors are best done when surrounded by a team of cheerleaders. As women, connection matters to us.

One of the longest studies ever done on health and happiness proved that positive relationships matter for our health. Harvard University launched an 80-year study starting in 1938 and ending in 2018 that tracked 268 Harvard graduates and more than 1,300 of their grandchildren hoping to see trends of what built a healthy and happy life. The conclusion? Tending to your relationships matters most to your health. According to the researchers' findings, tending to our relationships is a form of self-care. Subjects who maintained warm relationships lived longer, happier lives. Those who were lonelier died sooner. The head of the study, Dr. Robert Waldinger, a professor of psychiatry at Harvard Medical School, even went on to say, "Loneliness kills. It's as powerful as smoking or alcoholism."

Human connection is pivotal to your health. When you gather your community and engage in a group activity like this reset, you are setting yourself up for a great hormonal high. There are lots of ways you can build community around you. Start a book club, ask a friend to join you in these 30 days, or come find my free online communities. If you feel alone right now, please know that you are not. There is a world of like-minded women out there building a fasting lifestyle just like you who are ready to cheer you on. Lean in to them.

WHO IS THIS RESET FOR?

Honestly, it's for every woman. Having said that, because of the structure of this reset, it's great for women who are new to fasting and want to learn how to build a fasting lifestyle timed to their cycle. This reset is also fabulous for women without a cycle. It is an incredibly effective path to mastering fasting for women of all ages.

Although there are numerous health benefits to this reset, here are some of the symptoms and conditions that it helps the most:

- Weight-loss resistance
- Insulin resistance
- Diabetes
- Prediabetes
- Cardiovascular conditions
- Autoimmune conditions
- Memory problems
- Mood disorders such as anxiety and depression
- Hormonal cancers
- Infertility challenges
- Gut dysbiosis
- Menopause symptoms
- Brain fog
- Low energy
- Missed cycles
- Detoxing from birth control
- Repairing your gut post antibiotic use
- Lack of motivation
- Hair loss
- Thyroid challenges
- Accelerated aging

As always, it is best to collaborate with your doctor and advise him or her of this new fasting lifestyle you are about to embark upon.

PRE-RESET: TWO WEEKS LEADING UP TO YOUR 30-DAY FASTING RESET

If you have never fasted before, don't worry. This pre-reset is for you. Think of it as time to prepare your body for the fasting experience that is to come. I realize that you may have been eating six meals a day or indulging in many of the foods the Western diet provides. Jumping into a 17-hour fast with a dramatic food change could provide a strong stress response that makes you feel pretty crummy. Doing the pre-reset is a beautiful way to ease your body into the lifestyle changes you are about to make. If you are new to fasting, it takes about two weeks to prepare yourself for this 30-day experience. This is the right amount of time to see your blood sugar begin to come down, making it easier to move into a fasted state. Taking your time and setting yourself up with this pre-reset so that you succeed with your new fasting lifestyle is key. There are three easy parts to the pre-reset: foods to avoid, foods to add in, and compressing your eating window.

Foods to avoid

Here's the irony. Even though there is great scientific evidence that you can fast and then eat whatever you want and still get a great result, I encourage you to mind your food choices. Avoiding three food groups will make your 30-day experience much smoother. Your body will be ready to metabolically switch for 30 days. This will help you see quicker results in your 30-day reset, such as weight loss, energy boosts, and improved mental clarity.

The first category of foods to avoid are the bad oils that cause your cells to inflame and make you insulin resistant. They also often make you hungrier, which can easily derail your fasting efforts. In order to best avoid these oils, you are going to want to read ingredient labels. You might even have some of these oils in your house. If possible, I highly recommend you throw them out and replace them with healthier options like olive, avocado, and MCT oil.

The harmful oils you want to avoid are:

- Partially hydrogenated oils
- Corn oil
- Cottonseed oil
- Canola oil
- Vegetable oil
- Soybean oil
- Safflower oil
- Sunflower oil

You will also want to avoid refined sugars and flours. These foods are higher on the glycemic index and will put you on an up-and-down blood sugar roller coaster that can also make fasting harder. Removing them now will minimize any cravings you may get as you swap out inflammatory foods for healthy foods.

Foods high in refined flours and sugars include:

- Breads
- Pastas
- Crackers
- Desserts

When it comes to refined flours, women will often ask me about gluten-free flours. Many women are discovering that their bodies don't do well with gluten, the protein found in wheat grains. For some women, gluten can cause brain fog, weight gain, loss of energy, and a whole host of digestive problems. Although removing gluten from a product can help both your gut and brain, many gluten-free foods still spike your blood sugar and should be avoided during both the pre-reset and the 30-day reset itself. The other question I get is about sweeteners such as honey or coconut sugar. Although they are healthier options, these two ingredients should also be avoided during this time.

The third group of foods to remove are the ones filled with chemicals. These are the toxic ingredients I mentioned in Chapter 6. Many of these chemicals make you insulin resistant, which ultimately will make your fasting experience really hard. Because of their insulin resistance capabilities, these chemicals are often referred to as obesogens. Commonly found obesogens are high-fructose corn syrup, monosodium glutamate, and sugar substitutes like NutraSweet. NutraSweet, for example, can spike both glucose and insulin, and can stimulate the hunger centers in your brain. This is not the optimal environment you are looking for to thrive with your fasting lifestyle.

Common synthetic ingredients to avoid:

- Artificial colors and flavorings

- Red or blue dyes

- Saccharin

- NutraSweet

- Splenda

Foods to add

As you begin to remove some of the harmful foods that you have been eating for years, you may notice an uptick in unwanted cravings. This often happens for two reasons. One, because processed foods can feed bad microbes in your gut that control your cravings, as you pull these foods out of your diet, microbes often scream at you for more food. It can take up to three days for them to stop yelling at you. Two, these inflammatory foods often put your blood sugar on a roller-coaster ride, and when you remove them, it takes a couple of days for your blood sugar to even out. The best way to stop these cravings is to stabilize your blood sugar and kill your hunger hormones. This can be accomplished by adding more good fats and protein into your diet.

Good fats to add:

- Olive oil
- Avocado oil
- MCT oil
- Flaxseed oil
- Pumpkin seed oil
- Grass-fed butter
- Nut butters
- Olives
- Avocados

Healthy proteins to add:

- Grass-fed beef
- Bison
- Turkey
- Chicken
- Pork
- Eggs

- Charcuterie meats like salami and prosciutto

Compressing your eating window

During this time, you want to start to train your body for fasting. We call it compressing your eating window. At the start of this two-week period, move your breakfast back an hour. If you normally eat breakfast at 7 A.M., push it back to 8 o'clock. Every two days, push your breakfast another hour—9 A.M., then 10 A.M., etc.—until you can successfully go 13 hours without food. Once you can do that, you are ready for your 30-Day Fasting Reset. If you want to push your dinner back an hour and breakfast up an hour until you hit that 13-hour mark, that's okay as well. For example, if you normally finish dinner at 8 P.M. and eat breakfast at 6 A.M., you could finish your dinner at 7 P.M. and not eat breakfast until 8 A.M. This would give you a 13-hour fasting window.

You might be wondering what you can drink in your fasting window as you are training your body to adapt to this new eating schedule. This is when coffee and tea can really work to your advantage. Coffee and tea with a small amount of MCT oil and a clean cream can work to kill hunger and help you elongate your fasting period. MCT oil specifically helps your body switch over to fat-burning mode and will switch off the hunger hormone. If you like cream in your coffee, make sure it doesn't have any chemicals or sugar in it as this will spike your blood sugar too much and set you up for a difficult fasting experience.

Think of the pre-reset as a warm-up for your main fasting event. Once you have taken the first step to becoming a fat burner, I encourage you to go immediately into the 30-day reset.

TIPS FOR SUCCEEDING AT YOUR RESET

As I mentioned above, if you are new to fasting make sure you do the two-week pre-reset. This will make your 30-day reset much easier. Outside of doing the pre-reset, there are several other considerations I encourage you to think about.

First, remove the foods from your home and office that tempt you the most—anything that could derail you. One of my favorite foods is dried mangoes. I could eat bags of them all day long if I let myself. But any dried fruit, especially tropical fruit, is incredibly high on the glycemic index, so eating the whole bag was not in my best metabolic interest. As sad as it was, eventually I had to stop buying them. For me, it wasn't safe to have them in the house.

My second piece of advice is to remove the naysayers. I realize this is easier said than done, but I want you to surround yourself with people who cheer you on through this process, not bring you down. Your positive changes can often feel threatening to those around you who are stuck with their own health. Try to tune them out, or at least interact with them less during this 30-day experience. If misery loves company, so does positivity. Find yourself some positive people to hang out with during this time.

Also watch out for food buddies: those women you have bonded with over food. You know what I mean: We have had a bad day, so we call a friend and complain, and our friend offers to come over with a box of pizza and tub of ice cream to console us. No doubt these are fun friend moments. Although they feel good in the moment, they set us up for more miserable health days ahead. Years ago, I had an employee who went on an incredible weight-loss journey. As part of her new health regime, she started spending more time at the gym and less time at Starbucks with her friends drinking Frappuccinos. Eventually her friends became disgruntled and critical. Their lack of compassion ultimately derailed her efforts and eventually she gained all her weight back. If this resonates with you, encourage these women to do the reset with you or tell them that they'll just have to miss you for the next 30 days.

When to Start Your Reset

Outside of starting on day one of your cycle, I encourage you to also look at your social calendar before starting the reset. Have any weddings or vacations coming up? This is where women can derail their progress. Temptation can be high anywhere that there is plenty of food around. Having said that, once you get the hang of this reset, you will see fasting like a girl fits into the busiest of lives.

THE 30-DAY FASTING RESET

Whenever I start a new health program, I like to see the big picture of what I am doing first; then my mind is more receptive to the details. With that in mind, let's get a general overview of what your 30-day reset will look like and then go into the details.

There are three ground rules to remember as you move through this reset: You will avoid four major food categories, use two different eating styles, and experience three different fasting lengths.

OVERVIEW

Avoid

- Bad oils

- Refined flours and sugar
- Toxic chemical ingredients
- Alcohol

Food styles

- Ketobiotic
- Hormone feasting

Types of fasting

- Intermittent fasting (13 hours and 15 hours)
- Autophagy fasting (17 hours)

With the ground rules in place, let's walk through what your 30-Day Fasting Reset will look like. Remember, this reset is designed to help you metabolically shift in a way that maximizes your hormone production, so you will want to follow each day as it is laid out. The fasting length is what moves the most with this reset, especially in the power phases, so be sure you keep a close watch as to how long you should be fasting each day. Here is a day-to-day guide to your 30-day reset:

POWER PHASE 1

Food choice throughout the phase: ketobiotic
Days 1–4: intermittent fasting (13 hours)
Day 5: intermittent fasting (15 hours)
Days 6–10: autophagy fasting (17 hours)

MANIFESTATION PHASE

Food choice throughout the phase: hormone feasting foods
Days 11–15: intermittent fasting (13 hours)

POWER PHASE 2

Food choice throughout the phase: ketobiotic
Days 16–19: intermittent fasting (15 hours)

NURTURE PHASE

Food choice throughout the phase: hormone feasting
Days 20–30: no fasting

ADVANCED FASTING RESET

If you have been fasting for some time, follow this advanced version of the 30-day reset below. Longer fasts are here to stretch you and provide you with just enough hormetic stress to encourage your body to make that jump to the next level of health. You will also see that this reset gives you the option to fast the week before your cycle, if you have one. Because this is an advanced reset, the assumption is a shorter fast like 13 hours won't create a cortisol spike for you since your body is most likely used to this length of fast.

POWER PHASE 1-ketobiotic food

Days 1–5: intermittent fasting (15 hours)
Day 6: gut-reset fast (24 hours)
Days 7–10: autophagy fasting (17 hours)

MANIFESTATION PHASE-hormone feasting foods

Days 11–15: intermittent fasting (15 hours)

POWER PHASE 2-ketobiotic food

Day 16: gut-reset fast (24 hours)
Days 17–19: autophagy fasting (17 hours)

NURTURE PHASE-hormone feasting foods

Days 20–30: intermittent fasting (13 hours)

Tools to keep you on track

Remember that this reset is dynamic and there is much to monitor with your body. There are a few tools that can help you know what is going on as you fast, which can be very beneficial to your success. Now, I am not one to shill products, but one of the blessings this modern world has given us is the ability to self-check our biometrics. Biometrics are statistical analysis of key functions of your body. Blood pressure is a great example of a biometric. Your temperature would be another example of a common biometric. Old-school health used to have us going to our doctors all the time to get our biometric statistics. With the emergence of personalized health care, these tools are readily available to us at home to help us understand what is going on inside our bodies. These tools range in price, so I do want to emphasize that you can do this reset without them. Thousands of women in my community do. If you do have the resources to purchase them, they can be very helpful.

One of my favorite tools for fasters is monitoring your blood sugar and ketones. Diabetics have been measuring these two metrics on themselves for years. Now you can measure them too. I highly encourage you to get to know a tool called a glucose monitor. There are two types I recommend: finger test and continuous blood sugar readers. The finger test is where you prick your finger and put a drop of blood on a small stick that measures your blood sugar and ketones. A continuous glucose monitor is a device that typically goes into the back of your arm and gives you a continual reading of what your blood sugar is doing. Both have upsides and downsides. In Appendix C, I have listed my favorite versions of both tools.

These monitors provide three readings that are crucial for your success. The first is your morning reading. When you get up in the morning in a fasted state, take a blood glucose and ketone reading right away—before your coffee. You want your blood sugar to be in the range of 70–90 mg/dL (milligrams per deciliter). For most, your ketones will be low in the morning, possibly measuring at .2 mmol/L (millimoles per liter). You are in ketosis if you are over .5 mmol/L. The second reading to pay attention to is right before you eat your first meal of the day. You want to see that your blood sugar is lower than your morning reading and that your ketones are elevating. This means that in a fasted state your body is moving into fat-burning mode. The presence of ketones indicates you are now getting energy from the fat-burning energy system.

Let's look at a real-life example. Let's say you wake up at 7 A.M. and your readings are 98 mg/dL for your blood sugar and .1 mmol/L for ketones. Right before you break your fast a few hours later, you want to see your blood sugar go down below 98 mg/dL and your ketones go up above .1 mmol/L. If this switch happens, your body is trying to fat adapt. Even if that second ketone reading is not above .5 mmol/L, if it moves closer to that number your body is trying to switch over to fat burning. Small wins lead to big wins, so keep at your fasting lifestyle and you will eventually see those ketones go above .5 mmol/L.

The third reading you can take is two hours after you eat. Usually this is a blood sugar reading only, not ketones. This reading will help you see how well your meal did for your blood sugar. If you break your fast at noon and your blood sugar reading was at 78 mg/dL before you ate, two hours after that meal take another reading and see if your blood sugar is back down close to 78 mg/dL. If it is, then there is a great chance you are what we call insulin sensitive. Congrats! If it's not close to that original number, don't despair; the more you practice moving in and out of different-length fasts, the more you train your body to become insulin sensitive again.

Knowing how your blood sugar and ketones respond to this reset can be incredibly motivating and help you keep your focus. It is a more accurate measurement of how well you burn fat than the scale. If you have the resources to get a monitor, I highly encourage you to purchase one and use it.

As you get ready to embark upon your 30-day reset, there is one thing I want you to remember: Have compassion for yourself. Don't beat yourself up for making a mistake or slipping one day. That sort of negative talk will only discourage you. This should be fun. Be curious about what your body will do during each new fasting length. Enjoy learning these two new food styles. Experiment with what you like to break your fast with the most. The body will heal more quickly when you approach this process with joy and excitement for the journey. If you get stuck, lean in to community, look for the cheerleaders around you, and know you are not alone. I'm cheering you on!

CHAPTER 9

How to Break a Fast

To eat or not to eat—some people think fasting is that simple. But as you have read by now, fasting is a bit more complicated, and that goes for how to properly stay in a fast and how to properly end a fast. For something that takes only a second, there is a lot to think about. That is why I wanted to dedicate a whole chapter to how to break a fast.

As with many scientific discoveries, there has been an evolution of how we think about the art of fasting. When fasting first gained popularity, much of the focus was placed on the healing that was taking place while in the fasted state. Yet one huge question has not been addressed: Do those changes stick around once you eat again? Believe it or not, the research on food intake after your fast has not been very robust. As someone who loves to let the science guide me, I was left with little to go on and decided to do my own research. I turned to my community to see what worked best. After testing a variety of ways to break a fast on thousands of people, I have found there are four ways to approach the first bite of food you take after you've been fasting for several hours. How you determine which one of these styles is best for you depends on your health goals. Just like you choose your fasting length based on the healing effect you desire, you want to strategically break your fast to amplify the outcome you want.

RESET YOUR MICROBIOME

Think of fasting as the ultimate microbiome repair. When in a fasted state, you are giving the good bacteria in your gut a chance to thrive. You can continue to grow these helpful microbes by breaking your fast with one of the three Ps I spoke of in Chapter 6. The first P includes your probiotic-rich foods. These foods add good bacteria to your gut, so it makes a great food to break your fast with if you have been on multiple rounds of antibiotics or years of birth control. The second P, prebiotic foods, will feed your good microbes, so they make a great addition to a break-fast meal if you are wanting to grow more microbes that boost your immune system, provide yourself with more mood-enhancing neurotransmitters, or break down estrogen. The last P, polyphenol foods, are fabulous for repairing the mucosal lining of your gut; make sure you lean in to these foods if you have low energy, chronic pain, or brain fog from a leaky gut.

You can definitely combine all three of the Ps for a great breakfast meal. One of my favorite meals to break a fast with is half an avocado and a cup of sauerkraut sprinkled with pumpkin seeds and drizzled with flaxseed oil, hitting all the necessary components to grow good bacteria.

Foods to break your fast with that support your microbiome:

- Fermented yogurts, including coconut and dairy varieties
- Bone broth
- Sauerkraut
- Kombucha
- Seeds and seed oils
- Prebiotic-rich protein powders

BUILD MORE MUSCLE

A common misconception about fasting is that it breaks down muscle. I strongly disagree with this theory. Although it appears as if your muscles shrink when you fast, it's a temporary effect. Your muscles are releasing stores of sugar when you fast, causing them to appear smaller. This is a really good thing, because you can follow up that fast with a good protein punch and you will build your muscles stronger than ever. Think of fasting and eating protein as waves of an ocean. When you fast it's like a wave retracting so that it can gain momentum. When you eat, especially protein, you give that wave power to surge forward.

One of my favorite studies on protein showed that the most efficient way to stimulate mTOR was by eating 25 grams of protein every two hours.[1] Remember, 30 grams is what triggers an amino acid response in your muscles that encourages them to grow stronger. In this particular study, researchers found that periodic doses of 30 grams of protein cycled throughout the day was the most efficient way to build muscle. This makes protein a great macronutrient to break your fast with.

Many of the women I work with are over 40. After 40, as a woman goes through her perimenopause years, she often has to fight to maintain or build muscle. One strategy I love for these women is to have them work out in a fasted state, especially with a strength-training session, then follow up that workout with a protein-rich meal. This fasting-refeeding trick is one of the best I have seen for women who want to build muscle.

Protein comes in many forms. For meat eaters, my go-to suggestions for breaking a fast with protein are bone broth, eggs, or a sausage. If you eat a plant-based diet, your favorite protein shake may be the perfect meal to break your fast with. Many foods have protein in them, so you will have to experiment with what works best for you.

Foods to break your fast with that support muscle building:

- Eggs

- Beef sticks

- Beef jerky

- Protein shakes such as pea, hemp, and whey concentrate

- Sliced deli meats (nitrite-free)

- Chicken breast

- Turkey

- Grass-fed beef

- High-protein vegetables such as peas, broccoli, sprouts, mushrooms, and brussels sprouts

- Chickpeas

- Lima beans

- Quinoa

- Avocado

KEEP BURNING FAT

Of all the macronutrients, fat stabilizes your blood sugar the most. In fact, in many cases I have seen fats lower a person's blood sugar. This makes fats the perfect fuel to break a fast with if you are trying to elongate a fast to burn more fat. I have even used this trick with new fasters I've coached. If 13 hours seems like a daunting amount of time to go without food, eating a little fat during your fasting window often won't pull you out of a fasted state.

The hardest part is figuring out which fats to eat. *Fat bombs*, foods that are primarily made up of fat, is a term you hear followers of the ketogenic diet talk a lot about. Dreaming up new fat bombs can be challenging. The good news is that once you start looking for fat bombs you will notice that there are several companies that have created the perfect on-the-go fat bombs already. One of my favorites is called Keto Cups. You can always find these in my cupboards when I need a quick bite to eat but don't want to step out of ketosis. On my busiest workdays I often grab a couple of those to keep me going until I can sit down and have a proper meal. MCT oil in your coffee is another example of an added fat that helps during fasting. I have even seen people turn their coffee into a smoothie, adding grass-fed cream, butter, and MCT oil. If you put a little bit of prebiotic fibers in there, you'll also support the changing microbiome that fasting offers you.

Although I have fat listed here as breaking a fast, it technically doesn't break your fast; it just helps you lengthen your fasting time. As with all foods, you need to check it with your blood sugar to see what it does for you. Most people do notice that fat kills their hunger, but what it does to your blood sugar will depend on the variables I mentioned above.

Foods to break your fast with that keep you burning fat:

- Avocado
- Raw nuts or nut butter
- Olives
- Bone broth

FOLLOW YOUR TASTE BUDS

What happens if you make a poor food choice? Will you undo the good you did by fasting? The answer is no. Often new fasters will break their fast with whatever they want. Although this doesn't undo the healing effect of your fast, over time you will notice that it feels better to be intentional with what you break your fast with. I call this style of breaking a fast "following your taste buds." There are pros and cons to this approach. The only pro to this is instant satisfaction. The con is that all the healing effects of your fast will immediately stop once you dive into your favorite snacks, some of which may be pro-inflammatory. Easing out of your fast with one of the other three ways is always the best choice for your health. Having said that, science has shown us that a daily fasting regime of 14 to 16 hours will undo the metabolic damage poor diet can create in your body. You haven't lost the healing that happened while fasting, but this approach would be analogous to putting in a few hours at the gym and then going home and eating a tub of ice cream. Although the ice cream will raise your glucose and insulin, it won't negate the good your workout did. If you have specific health goals that you are trying to achieve, no doubt this approach will slow your progress. The same is true with fasting. If you break your fast with junk food, it doesn't undo the good you did while fasting; it just might not get you to your health destination as quickly as you would like.

Can you see why I wanted to dedicate a whole chapter to breaking a fast? It's not as simple as "do this; don't do that." There are many things to consider. One reason I wanted to help you see the factors that affect blood sugar regulation is that I have watched thousands of women get frustrated with fasting largely because they don't understand the nuance of blood sugar. This is such an important point. I never want you to be discouraged with your fasting efforts at the expense of a lack of knowledge. It's easy to get frustrated when you can't move into ketosis, even when you feel like you are doing all the right steps. If this is ever you, revisit this chapter and remind yourself of the small details that may matter to your blood sugar.

WHAT PULLS YOU OUT OF A FASTED STATE?

This is where it gets personal. You are fasting but need something—anything—to get you through the next few hours. Now, there are things that you can drink that won't pull you out of the fast, but it really depends on your own body—and your blood sugar response. Remember, it takes about eight hours after your last meal to begin to make this switch. If your blood sugar elevates at all during this time, it will switch you back to your sugar-burner system. If you want to stay in a fasted state, the name of the game is to keep your blood sugar low. Anything that causes your blood sugar to rise will pull you out of your fast, whether you want it to or not. Having said that, there are some drinks you can have in your fasting window that will not raise your blood sugar, and therefore won't pull you out of your fasted state. Although you need to always test these drinks with the blood sugar test I give you below, the most common drinks that fasters use in their fasting window are coffee, tea, and mineral water.

What breaks a fast for you may not break a fast for me. You need to be your own n of 1 and test. In general, there are two major variables that will affect how your blood sugar reacts in a fasted state: the diversity of your microbiome and your degree of insulin resistance. It would be a whole lot easier for me to just say tea will break your fast and coffee won't, but because of our bio-individuality it's not that simple. Understanding these two variables will be helpful to customize fasting to your body.

Poor microbial diversity

The diversity of your microbiome has a huge influence over how your blood sugar will respond to the foods and drinks you consume. A healthy, diverse microbiome leads to better blood sugar management. I experienced this firsthand. When I first wore a continuous glucose monitor, my blood sugar would elevate pretty dramatically every time I ate a protein-rich meal. Luckily, within two hours it returned to its premeal level, giving me an indication that I had good insulin sensitivity, but the high spike surprised me. Knowing the impact that the microbiome has on blood sugar regulation, I focused on improving my gut microbiome for several months using many of the fasting and food hacks I have taught you here. Three months later, I put another continuous glucose monitor on. This time when I ate protein, my blood sugar dropped. Same protein, different microbiome diversity. That's how powerful your microbiome is to blood sugar regulation.

What's the mechanism behind how these microbes regulate your blood sugar? Well, it turns out that your gut microbes have a direct connection to your liver via your portal vein.[2] When in a fasted state, these microbes will send a signal to the liver to switch over to the fat-burning energy system. If these microbes are missing, then that signal may never get to the liver, making it difficult for you to stay in a fasted state. I see this a lot in women who have been on multiple rounds of antibiotics and have lost much of their microbial diversity. They will struggle to get into ketosis because these missing microbes aren't sending signals to the liver to switch over.

The good news is you can repair your microbiome quickly—some experts believe in a matter of days. If your coffee elevates your blood sugar today, as you repair your microbiome that response may change.

Insulin resistance

If your cells are insulin resistant, you will notice a spike in blood sugar with even the most benign of drinks. I have seen a glass of water raise a person's blood sugar if they are severely insulin resistant. Yet there are varying degrees of insulin resistance. You don't have to be diagnosed with diabetes to be insulin resistant. There is a spectrum. If you are not getting into ketosis easily or are feeling like everything is pulling you out of a fasted state, you may be more insulin resistant than you realize. Keep working on your fasting lifestyle, and with time this resistance will go away. Knowing these two factors can be very helpful in determining what drinks or possibly morsel of food is best to have while fasting.

Blood Sugar Test

There is a very easy way to test what pulls you out of a fasted state. You get a blood sugar reader and take just the glucose reading. Once you have that as a baseline, drink the drink that you are curious about and then take another reading half an hour later. If those two readings are the same or the second reading is lower than the first, you are still in a fasted state. If that second reading is higher than the first, it's pulled you out of a fasted state and put you back into a sugar-burner state. I tell people to test their morning cup of coffee first, because coffee affects everyone's blood sugar differently; it's to know how it impacts your fasted state. This test also helps you determine whether your body does well with some of the common coffee additions such as cream, MCT oil, butter, and stevia.

Having said that, after watching thousands of people fast, there are generally drinks that will work while you are fasting and ones that I can tell you with certainty should not be in your fasting window.

Things that often pull you out of a fasted state:

- Coffee creamers

- Sweeteners in your coffee or tea

- Sodas

- Diet drinks

- Gatorade

- Alcohol

Things that don't typically pull you out of a fasted state:

- Supplements
- Medications
- Black coffee
- Coffee with full-fat milk
- Tea
- Oils, including flaxseed and MCT
- Mineral water

Fasted snack

Is there ever a time when you can eat during your fasted state without breaking your fast? It's possible with a fasted snack, which can be a really helpful tool to utilize if need be, especially when you are first learning to fast. Research actually shows that people who use a fasted snack are able to elongate their fasting windows and lose more weight.[3] Identifying which fasted snack works best for you can be tricky, so make sure you test it with your blood sugar. Some fats that I have seen work as a fasted snack for some women are nut butter, bone broth, or even coffee powered up with full-fat cream and butter. Just remember that once you get to a place where you don't need that fasted snack, stop having it. Use fasted snacks as a crutch only as you get used to the longer fasts.

Good fasted snacks:

- ¼ cup of grass-fed cream
- 1 tablespoon of MCT oil
- 2 tablespoons of nut butter
- 1 tablespoon of seed oil

Breaking Longer Fasts

When you do shorter fasts (less than 48 hours), you want to lean in to the therapeutic strategies I mentioned above. If you choose to do a fast that's longer than 48 hours, then you'll want to stick to the following formula.

Why is that? Forty-eight hours or longer without food is long enough for your digestion to slow down significantly. This means that when you reintroduce food, you want to be strategic about how you do that. The first three-day water fast I went on, I was so excited to eat food that I had a huge plate of scrambled eggs afterward. I immediately felt sleepy. I also felt like I had a huge lump in my stomach, and it took almost 24 hours for that feeling to go away. To avoid this reaction, I came up with four steps to follow when you break a longer fast. These steps will ensure that you are refeeding your microbiome properly and easing back into food.

Step #1: Drink a cup of broth

You can choose any type of broth you want. I've already talked about bone broth as a great way to support your gut. Bone broth has glycine in it and can heal a leaky gut. If you know you have some gut healing to do, this is a great broth to break your fast with for added gut repair. If you are vegetarian, vegetable broth works well too.

Think of this cup of broth as a warm-up to food. Your digestion has been shut off for several days, so introducing solid food can be difficult. After you drink a cup of broth, wait an hour before you move to step two.

Step #2: Eat a probiotic-rich meal with fat

After a three-day water fast, you have a real opportunity to refeed your good bacteria. Probiotic foods are the best way to do that. Much like the recommendation I gave above, after you do broth, add in some fermented yogurt or sauerkraut. Even a liquid fermented drink like kombucha works well at this point. I often will have a bowl of olives, which are rich in polyphenols, for added fat. Wait another hour after this step before you proceed to step three.

Step #3: Steam veggies

Now you are ready to try a little more fiber. This is the point at which you are going to gain some insight into your microbiome. If you hit this step and get bloated, you'll know that you have more gut repair to do. Be sure to add a few gut-reset fasts into your fasting lifestyle, followed by breaking your fast with the three Ps. This third step can be diagnostic for you, helping you see where to focus your health efforts next.

You don't want to do raw vegetables at this point because they have too much fiber and can be hard for your digestive system to break down. Lightly steamed vegetables will be easier on your digestive tract. You can drizzle some good oils on top and sprinkle some salt over your vegetables if you want for added taste. Another good food at this time is a small sweet potato. Sweet potatoes—especially purple sweet potatoes—feed the good bacteria in your lower intestinal tract. At this step I will often add some grass-fed butter and Himalayan sea salt to get good fats and minerals back in. Wait another hour before proceeding to step four.

Step #4: Ready to eat animal protein

Now your digestive system is ready for meat. If you want to build muscle, be sure to have at least 30 grams at this first meal; if you want to stay in autophagy, keep it under 20 grams. People commonly ask whether they can have a full meal at this point. The answer is yes. The first three steps were to prepare you for this meal. If you eat meat too early, it can be miserable. By the time you get to this point, you are ready to integrate most foods back in.

I hear a lot from women that they worry they will boomerang back into poor food choices after a long fast like this. If you have that same fear, this four-step process is your break-fast tool. It's a slow and methodical approach to a long healing fast that will ensure that you keep the healing effects of this fast for months to come.

Whatever method you choose to break your fast with, the key is to be intentional about that first food that goes in your mouth. The more you are strategic about how you break your fast, the quicker your health results will come.

Now that I have given you hacks for breaking your fast, let's look at some other general hacks that will level up your fasting game.

CHAPTER 10

Hacks That Make Fasting Effortless

I'm notoriously impatient, so I am always looking for the fastest (no pun intended) path to a result I can find. I also like to share, so I always impart new hacks with my community so that they, too, get more out of their own fasting journey.

I do have a word of caution for you, though. While these hacks often accelerate the healing process and help you avoid any unwanted detours, the goal of healing isn't always about speed (a lesson that I need to heed as well). So I ask you to keep three principles to healing in mind. The first is that healing takes time. Although fasting will yield you results quickly, if you have a chronic condition, it will take time to heal. Be patient. Trust your fasting process. The more you keep at your fasting lifestyle, the more opportunities you give your body for healing. The second principle is practice. If you were to learn a new instrument, you wouldn't be able to just pick up that instrument and start playing it perfectly, right? Well, like any worthwhile endeavor, it takes practice to start to get the hang of it. The same goes with fasting. It's a new tool. Be curious about it. Give yourself grace if you have days that are less than perfect. If you set out to do a 17-hour fast and make it only 13 hours, don't beat yourself up. I constantly tell my community that there is no such thing as a failed fast. Each day you fast you put yourself into a healing state. Keep at it and in time you will see a change. The last healing principle is to keep deepening your knowledge of how your body works. The more you understand why fasting works and learn about the miracle of why your body wants to metabolically switch, the better you'll integrate fasting into your life. On my YouTube channel, I often say, "Knowledge is your fuel." There is no doubt that the more you learn about fasting, the easier it will be to create a fasting lifestyle that is perfect for you.

So let me get you started on that road of knowledge. Below are the most common hacks my community uses to excel at their fasting lifestyle. Integrated into these hacks are answers to some of the more common questions I have received over the years. Read through them all and remember that they are here for you to return to for reference if you hit an obstacle at any point in your journey.

HANDLING HUNGER WHEN FASTING

Hunger is the elephant in the fasting room. Every faster has to learn how to navigate hunger. In fact, it's often the first question I get. Depending on how metabolically flexible you are, hunger can happen, but there are several great hacks for staving it off.

The first question to ask yourself is, "Am I hungry or am I bored?" It can be hard to tell sometimes. Food is an emotional state changer. Knowing the difference between boredom and hunger can be helpful. First do an activity that lifts your mood. Play your favorite song. Dance around your kitchen. Get a dose of oxytocin by calling your favorite friend. Watch a funny movie. Sometimes even taking a nap can help. Try elevating your mood with another tool other than food and see if the hunger goes away.

After you've acknowledged that you are truly hungry and not bored, the next go-to is a packet of minerals. Two of my favorites are put out by LMNT and Redmond. Hunger can be caused by many things, and sometimes it is triggered by a mineral imbalance. So get a boost of sodium, potassium, and magnesium. Not only do these packets have great flavors that satisfy your taste buds, but they dissolve easily in water, making them a great drink to sip on in your fasting window. And don't worry about your blood pressure spiking: If you ingest sodium when insulin is lower, it won't contribute to high blood pressure. Make sure the packets you use are unsweetened so they don't spike your blood sugar and take you out of a fasted state. On the days that I fast longer, I like to put a pack of minerals in a water bottle and sip on it all morning long.

Still hungry? If the first two hacks don't work, it may be time to lean in to a fasted snack. Remember the fasted snack? If you are extending your fast to 15 hours and your body is used to just 13 hours of fasting, a small fat bomb can often be the tool you need to make it two more hours. Sometimes a fat bomb can be as simple as full-fat cream and some MCT oil in your tea or coffee in the morning. This is what many fasters do. Since everyone's body responds differently to these fat bombs, test them with your blood sugar (as discussed in Chapter 9) to see if they work for your blood sugar. If so, then you might find it helpful to have a cup of coffee in the morning loaded with fat to help you make it to lunch without breaking your fast.

Lastly, one little-known hack is to feed your microbiome in a fasted state. What does this mean? Often it's not your human cells that are requesting food; your gut microbes are the ones screaming at you. If you feed those microbes, they stop giving you hunger signals. You can do this by adding a prebiotic powder to your water, coffee, or tea. Remember, prebiotics feed the good bacteria in your gut. Specifically, the prebiotic fiber inulin can appropriately nourish these little critters.

WHEN TO USE COFFEE AND TEA WHILE FASTING

Drinking a cup of coffee or mug of tea during your fasting window can be extremely helpful. But again, I would recommend testing it with your blood sugar. Coffee can stimulate autophagy, which is a great thing, but as I mentioned before, everyone reacts differently to coffee. One key concept to realize is that not all coffee is made alike. Many coffees are packed with pesticides and even have mold in them. It's these chemicals that can spike your blood sugar. Make sure your coffee is mold- and pesticide-free. Coffees that are free of these toxins will often say "organic" or "mold-free" on their packaging. When in doubt reach out to the company and ask. Many coffee shops are proud of their pure coffee, so look for cafés that publicly tout their pure offerings. Coffee that has a lot of chemicals in it will keep you insulin resistant, so avoid those chemical-laden coffees at all costs.

HANDLING DETOX SYMPTOMS

When you go into ketosis for the first few times, it's common to get something called the keto flu. Symptoms of the keto flu may include rashes, fevers, muscle aches, constipation, brain fog, and fatigue. No doubt these symptoms can be disturbing. And since we have been taught to medicate symptoms rather than interpret them, it's easy to villainize fasting for causing the symptomatic outburst. Remember that ketones will have a healing effect on your body, and when the body is healing it is often symptomatic. Think of the typical flu: Your body raises its temperature to burn an infection out. Or your body makes mucus to stick to viruses so that it can escort them out of your system. Rashes can appear as your body pushes bacteria and viruses out through your skin. These are all positive signs that the body is healing.

If you are experiencing strong detox symptoms, I recommend three things. First, make sure you are varying your fasts, much like the variation I provided for you with the 30-Day Fasting Reset. I find detox symptoms don't appear as frequently when you vary your fasts, especially if you skip a day or two of fasting and then come back to your fasting lifestyle. This gives your body a chance to catch up with the surge of toxins that might be pouring out of you.

The second trick is to be sure to open up your detox pathways so that toxins can effectively move through you. Weight gain can also be a sign of congested detox pathways. These pathways include your liver, gut, kidneys, lymph, and skin. Remember, fasting can have a detox effect to it, especially with fasts that are 17 hours or longer. When your body goes into a detox, it has to push toxins out through one of the above pathways.

There are several hacks for opening your detox pathways. Be sure to also look at my favorite liver hacks outlined below.

- **Dry brushing**
  Daily dry brushing with a special hard brush can exfoliate your skin and open up pores that allow toxins to exit your system.

- **Sweating**
  Sweating moves circulation and opens up pores, letting toxins out of your body. A good daily sweat can dramatically help fasting detox reactions.

- **Lymph massage**
  Your lymphatic system is what carries toxins away from your organs. If your lymph is stagnant, you might have more detox reactions than necessary. A good lymphatic massage can be helpful to get your lymph moving again.

- **Rebounder trampoline**
  Jumping up and down can also move the lymphatic system. A daily dose of rebounding on a trampoline can keep your lymph flowing.

- **Epsom salt bath**
  Warm water mixed with magnesium is magic for extracting toxins from your skin. This can be especially helpful for detox symptoms such as rashes, headaches, and joint pain.

The last trick is to use binders such as a zeolite or activated charcoal. Zeolites often come in a liquid form, and activated charcoal is usually found in a capsule. My favorite zeolite is CytoDetox by 180° Solution, whereas my go-to for activated charcoal is called BIND by Systemic Formulas. Remember, when you stimulate autophagy, unhealthy cells die, causing environmental toxins and heavy metals to be released into your system. Your body will push those toxins out through the skin, gut, and kidneys. Binders can help grab on to those toxins and get them out of you.

MEASURING BLOOD SUGAR AND KETONES

Measuring your blood sugar and ketones is entirely up to you. I find it helpful so that you can understand what your fasting lifestyle is doing for you. If you do decide to check them, the best time is first thing in the morning and right before your first meal. You want your blood sugar to be between 70 and 90 milligrams per deciliter (4.0–5.0 millimoles per liter) and your ketones over .5 mmol/L. You also want to see on your second reading that your blood sugar is dropping and your ketones are going up. This is a signal that your body is moving toward a fat-burner energy source.

There are many ways to look at blood sugar and ketones. There are two types of measurement tools I love and two that I would encourage you to stay away from. The two to avoid are the urine measurements and the breathalyzers. Both of these measurements have proven to be not only inaccurate but also hard to read. With urine, for example, it tells you only what the ketone load is exiting out of your body. It doesn't tell you what is readily available for your brain. To date, breathalyzers have proven to be hard to use and not always accurate.

The measurement tools that I do recommend are a blood sugar and ketone meter and a continuous glucose meter. The blood sugar and ketone meters are inexpensive and convenient to use. You prick your finger with a lancet that draws a small drop of blood. That drop goes on a small stick that is inserted into the meter. Fairly quickly you get a blood sugar and ketone reading. If you don't mind pricking your finger, it's a pretty easy tool to use. The continuous glucose monitor, also known as CGM, takes blood sugar readings to a whole new level. It will continuously measure your blood sugar so that you can get a reading of what foods work best for you. This tool is not only helpful for understanding how your blood sugar responds in a fasted state, but it's also helpful for seeing what impact a meal has on your blood sugar. Recently I did three days of 24-hour fasts followed by protein-only meals. I was surprised to learn that after a full day of fasting, a protein-rich meal actually dropped my blood sugar. I would have never guessed that if I hadn't had my continuous glucose meter on. I also like CGMs to determine whether your liver is dumping glucose in the middle of the night. With a moment-by-moment picture of your blood sugar you can gain so much insight about which foods and fasts work best for you.

Signs you are in ketosis

There are several ways to determine whether you are in ketosis. The first is by how you feel, and the second is by your ketone reader. You know you are in ketosis when you're not hungry, you have incredible mental clarity, and your energy is strong and steady. If you choose to use a ketone reader, you'll know you are in ketosis when the reader says .5 mmol/L or greater.

STRATEGIES FOR GETTING YOUR BLOOD SUGAR TO DECREASE

Often when you start building a fasting lifestyle, you will find that your blood sugar struggles to lower. This happens often when you are first training your body to be a fat burner. In fact, I tell all new fasters this is your first step: Get into ketosis. But what if you are doing all the right things and still not getting into ketosis? There are six hacks I recommend. You might have to try each one before you find the perfect fit for you.

Hack #1-Fast longer

You might need to fast longer. Recently a friend told me that fasting wasn't working for her weight-loss efforts. I asked her how long she was fasting, and she said 15 hours every day. I advised her to try a 36-hour fat-burner fast just one time and see what it did for her. Sure enough, that was the trick. She started losing weight for the first time in years. A little more hormetic stress flipped her metabolic switch and pushed her over to fat-burning mode. Sometimes your body just needs to play with these principles for a while before it can make that switch to the ketogenic fat-burning pathways. Hang in there. Your body knows what to do.

Hack #2-Vary your fasts

Variation confuses your neurology. When we get stuck in routines and habits, our body is no longer forced to adapt in positive ways. When the pandemic first hit, I had a packed schedule of seminars I was going to speak at. Within a matter of weeks, all of those seminars were canceled and I was stuck at home. Although not my first choice, I quickly fell in love with some simple pleasures like doing puzzles and tending to my garden. I also got great joy from watching the families in my neighborhood riding bikes together and enjoying each other's company. For a brief moment, this bizarre new world I was living in was strangely blissful. But six months later, like many of you I was agitated by my quarantine life. I no longer felt like it lifted me up and I was ready for a drastic change.

The same experience can happen to you when you stick to the same fasts. At first it can be miraculous. But if you don't vary your fasts, your body may stop adapting. This can show up as trouble getting into ketosis or getting your blood sugar to come down. Don't get stuck in the rut of doing only your favorite fast. Experiment with all six types of fasting. You might even need to throw in a few days when you don't fast. Then go back to fasting in order to make your cells more metabolically flexible.

Hack #3-Avoid ALL processed foods

Processed foods make you insulin resistant. Removing them from your diet can dramatically affect your ability to get into ketosis. Bad oils, refined sugars and flours, and chemicals make it hard to step out of being a sugar burner. I have seen many times where a person is doing all the right things with fasting but blocking their results by eating processed foods during their eating window. Remember the standard American diet is what is causing you to be insulin resistant and inflamed, and keeping you from your God-given fat-burning capabilities. The big three insults to your health are oils, sugar, and chemicals. Mind them carefully.

Hack #4-Love your liver

Your liver is the hardest-working organ in your body. It might need some love in order to move you into ketosis. Your liver is what senses the decrease in blood sugar and makes the switch over to the ketogenic fat-burning pathways. If your liver is congested and not performing at its best, you may struggle to make this switch. Be sure to minimize habits that load the liver, like drug and alcohol use. I find that the liver is often the problematic organ that prevents people from going into ketosis. Not to mention that much of the sugar your body has stored over the years exists in your liver. A healthy liver is key for succeeding at your fasting lifestyle. The following are my favorite liver hacks.

- **Castor oil packs:** These are premade packs that you cover in organic castor oil and put over your liver for a minimum of two hours at a time three times a week. The castor oil helps dilate the common bile duct that is responsible for moving toxins out of the liver and gallbladder.

- **Coffee enemas:** These kits, which can be bought online, work to dilate the liver and common bile duct so that toxins move through that area more efficiently. One time a week is perfect for opening up your liver.

- **Infrared saunas:** These can induce a fever-like effect in your cells, encouraging them to burn out any pathogens or toxins that are disrupting the cell. Daily saunas can be key for opening up your pathways.

- **Essential oils:** Essential oils like mandarin orange, geranium, and rosemary are great for opening up liver detox pathways. Just a few drops on the skin over the liver after a hot shower or infrared sauna are all that is needed.

- **Bitter lettuces:** Bitter lettuces give your liver the necessary nutrients to function properly. Add them into your greens daily for extra liver support.

- **Dandelion tea:** A daily cup of organic dandelion tea can nourish a sluggish liver.

Hack #5-Support your adrenals

When your adrenals are fatigued, regulating your blood sugar can be challenging. If you are struggling to get into ketosis, it may be that your HPA (hypothalamic-pituitary-adrenal) axis is challenged. The first thing to know about adrenal fatigue is that your adrenals work like a team with your brain. A misconception is that the adrenals wear out, but that is not what is actually happening. Organs don't just mysteriously wear out. The challenge that often arises is that the communication from the brain to the adrenals is challenged. There are a couple of telltale signs that this connection between your brain and adrenals may be off. The first is when you go from sitting to standing and you get dizzy. Since your adrenals play a part in blood pressure, this can indicate that your adrenals were slow to react to the positional change. The other sign that your adrenals may be struggling is your craving for salt. You can run a DUTCH hormone test and see exactly what is going on with your adrenals. The other strategy is to jump into boosting your adrenals with supplementation.

Hack #6-Remove toxins

Remove toxins. If all the above tricks don't work, it might be time to look at your toxic load with long-standing toxins like heavy metals. Heavy metals stay stuck in your tissues for years and can make the liver sluggish, destroy mitochondria in your cells, and contribute to insulin resistance. If ketosis is not coming to you easily, it may be time to detox.

OPENING UP DETOX PATHWAYS TO IMPROVE WEIGHT LOSS

Keeping your detox pathways open when you fast is key for accelerating weight loss. If you gain weight when you're first starting out, you may think, *I must be doing something wrong*. But don't worry, there is a physiological reason why you might gain weight while fasting. Weight gain is a sign that one or more of your detox pathways—the liver, gut, kidneys, lymph, and skin —are congested. Remember, fasting can have a detox effect to it, especially fasts that are 17 hours or longer. When your body goes into a detox, it has to push toxins out through one of the above pathways. If your body is holding on to weight while you are fasting, there is a good possibility that one or more of these pathways is congested. Be sure you are having daily bowel movements, sweating often, drinking lots of water, dry brushing or loofah brushing your skin, placing castor oil packs over your liver at night, and getting lymphatic drainage massage on a monthly basis. Opening up these pathways will ensure your body doesn't continue to store any toxins in fat.

PREVENTING UNWANTED CYCLE CHANGES

Both spotting and missed cycles with otherwise normal menstrual periods can indicate low progesterone. If you are postmenopausal and start spotting out of nowhere, understand that this is not uncommon. Many times women go into menopause early because of environmental stressors. When these women come to fasting, the damage caused by those stressors is repaired, especially if autophagy is being stimulated. For postmenopausal women, this new spotting is usually not something to be concerned with; in fact, it's something to celebrate. Your body is healing in new ways.

"What if there is a long time in between my cycles?" I hear this a lot, especially from perimenopausal women. Go through a cycle as usual; when you get to day 30 of the reset and your period hasn't started yet, just start over again on day one and go another 30 days. As a perimenopausal woman, your cycles will be random. A couple of rounds of the 30-Day Fasting Reset often syncs your cycle back up again. Although ultimately as you move closer to your postmenopausal years your cycles will space out more and be shorter, if you are experiencing extreme symptoms of menopause or are moving into menopause earlier than is appropriate for your body, the 30-Day Fasting Reset can help. This is what happened to me in my late 40s as I worked these principles on myself. I thought I was heading into menopause around age 47, but since I have been following the principles of the Fasting Cycle, at 52 my cycle has been more predictable and regular.

FASTING AND SPECIFIC CONDITIONS

Fasting and hair loss

This is common yet avoidable. The modern world has us mineral depleted. You need minerals to keep your hair full and growing. My first solution to hair loss is to take a mineral supplement. If that doesn't help, be sure you vary your fasting lengths while avoiding fasts that are longer than 17 hours. It's at 17 hours that the toxic dump can begin.

If you have done both of the tips above and are still experiencing hair loss, consider getting a heavy metal test. Heavy metals like lead, mercury, and thallium will sit in mineral receptor sites of your cells and make it difficult for minerals to get in. Thallium in particular is prevalent in our oceans from the Fukushima nuclear fallout. This heavy metal is now in many of the fish we are eating. We have run thousands of heavy metal tests on women and have come to discover that those with the worst levels of thallium are also the ones with the worst hair loss.

Another toxic influx that seems to affect hair loss comes from the chemicals in breast implants. If you are thinking about getting implants, I would encourage you to do your research. Ask about the type of implants your doctor wants to use and find out what they are made of. If you already have implants, this is a tough conversation, I know. Many implants have heavy metals in them—find out if yours do. Once you know what's in them, you can make that difficult decision; it may behoove you to get them removed. If it helps, I have been in the detox trenches with a lot of very sick women and the ones who have had their implants removed feel so much better and never regret the decision.

Fasting and fatigue

Remember that you are repairing your mitochondria with your fasting lifestyle. That means that initially you can get a little fatigued. My first recommendation is to give yourself permission to be tired. Can you go to bed early, take a quick, 20-minute power nap, or just sit and rest for a few? You are healing, and it takes energy from your cells to heal. If the low energy persists, this is where you might lean in to some biohacking tools that help power up your mitochondria. One is red light therapy. Your mitochondria have receptors on the outside of their membranes for red light; this therapy provides them with necessary light fuel and allows them to provide you with energy. Another biohack is a hyperbaric oxygen chamber. Your cells require oxygen to function normally, yet as you age your cells become less efficient at taking the oxygen you breathe in and putting it into your cells. A hyperbaric oxygen chamber compresses oxygen so that it can get into your cells and feed your mitochondria. If the fatigue with fasting lasts for several weeks, it might be time to detox. Environmental toxins destroy mitochondria function. If fasting isn't energizing those powerhouses, removing toxins from your cells will help them perform better.

Fasting and medications

I also get asked a lot about medications while fasting. All medications will respond differently when you fast, and if you take any medication, you will want to involve your doctor in your fasting decisions. I have seen thyroid medication, in particular, respond uniquely to a fasting window. As you fast you might be more sensitive to your thyroid medication; your heart rate may rise or you may feel like you are getting a thyroid storm. Because of this I would recommend taking your medication during your eating window or with your buttered coffee in the morning. I also highly recommend talking to your doctor, letting him or her know you are doing more fasting and might need some adaptations as to when and how much thyroid medication you take.

Fasting and supplements

Can you take your supplements during your fasting window? In general the answer is yes. It's a preference. If you can take supplements on an empty stomach, go for it. If that makes you feel nauseated, then I recommend taking them during your eating window. I have seen B vitamins cause stomach issues when fasting. If you take a supplement with B vitamins in it and notice some nausea afterward, try taking the supplement during your eating window instead.

One caveat: I would not recommend taking supplements during a three-day water fast. When we are trying to make systemic stem cells, it's best to just let the intelligence of your body sort things out. When you take supplements during those longer fasts, they can alter the healing reactions that kick in when fasting.

Fasting and cravings

Cravings often come from changes in your mineral balance and changes in your microbiome. Be sure you are supplementing with a good mineral supplement. Also know that your gut bacteria controls cravings too, and fasting will kill bad gut bacteria and help you grow good ones. Those bad bacteria will shout at you as they are dying off, often triggering cravings for chocolate, carbohydrates, or sugars. This is definitely the case with the fungus called candida, which makes you crave carbs and sugar in a big way. As you are starving it out with fasting, it can increase your cravings. Hang in there; the more you fast, the more those cravings will go away.

What to do when you fall off your fasting lifestyle

First, the key principle of fasting is that there is no such thing as a failed fast. If you struggle and fall off, just release any judgment you may have of yourself and hop right back on. Don't carry the guilt with you into the next day. The hardest part of letting yourself down and slipping backward with your fasting goals is forgiving yourself. All fasts help you, so release the guilt. Let it go and start anew the next day. Remember, each time you make an attempt at fasting it gets easier and easier. Look at it like you are training for a marathon. Each day you stretch your runs a little longer, you're building yourself stronger for the next workout. If you set out to run eight miles and you run only six miles, you are still in the process of training. Each time you "fail" at fasting and start again you move one step closer to building a fasting lifestyle that feels effortless to you.

Fasting and sleep

Two questions I hear a lot from fasters are why they can't sleep as much as they're used to, and why they have pain when they sleep. Some women find they require less sleep when they fast, especially with fasts that are longer than 24 hours. At first this symptom can feel a little disturbing, but when you break down what happens to you when you sleep and when you fast, you will see that they are both healing states. Your body repairs when you sleep. This is the main part of your 24-hour cycle that it does this. When you add fasting into that 24-hour cycle, you are repairing as well. Your body might decide it needs less sleep. This tends to happen with a longer fast like a three-day water fast. There not much to do about this symptom except to honor that it's happening and perhaps even take advantage of it: If you wake up earlier in the morning, try journaling, meditating, or reading a book. So much insight happens when we fast. Use those early morning hours to fuel your spiritual practice.

The other common sleep symptom I see with fasters is aches and pains showing up at night, typically on three-day water fasts. Women often complain of pelvic and low-back pain. Because of the stem cell production that happens during longer fasts, your body may be repairing scar tissue that was damaged from carrying and delivering babies. We don't often think of the residual physical effects of pregnancy, but our bodies do, and those stem cells go to areas that need the most repair. There are a few tricks to help ease the pain: One, increase your magnesium before you go to bed to relax your muscles. It also will help you sleep more soundly. Two, try CBD, in either a lotion over the painful areas or as a tincture. There is great scientific evidence that CBD can turn off pain receptors—and it's natural with no side effects.

Fasting and exercise

Working out in a fasted state during shorter fasts can be a helpful weight-loss tool. Your body will naturally elevate its blood sugar during exercise in order to meet the physical demands of the workout. Remember, the first three places your body will store extra blood sugar are your liver, muscles, and fat. Often your body will metabolize fat much quicker when you work out fasted. Post-workout, break your fast with protein and you'll develop a lean, muscular look.

I do not, however, recommend working out while doing a three-day water fast. What you are doing when you enter this length of fast is asking your body to go into a massive repair state. Much like you wouldn't work out when you have a fever, which is a healing state, I recommend halting all exercise when you do this fast. Give your body a chance to go into full repair mode.

Fasting after a hysterectomy

Anyone who has had a surgical procedure that has changed or ended their cycle abruptly will benefit from the 30-Day Fasting Reset. After a surgery like a hysterectomy, your body will still make sex hormones. Your adrenals are one part of the body that will help give you some of this hormonal juice. Since the 30-day reset is meant to help you maximize sex hormone production, following the steps of this reset will help support the remaining tissues.

Fasting with a thyroid condition

Your thyroid needs five organs to work properly: the brain, thyroid, liver, gut, and adrenals. Every cell in your body has a receptor site for thyroid hormones, so the other key part of the thyroid equation is that you need your cells to be free from toxins and inflammation. Knowing all the organ players involved in your thyroid condition can be helpful.

Here is a simplistic overview of how your body makes and uses your thyroid hormones. Your brain, specifically the pituitary gland that sits at the base of the skull, will release TSH (thyroid stimulating hormone), which travels down to the thyroid and activates it to make a hormone called thyroxine, or T4. This hormone will travel to the liver and gut to get converted into a hormone called triiodothyronine, or T3, the version of your thyroid hormones that is to be used by your cells. T3 will travel to a cell and move into it via a receptor site so that it can be put to use. The one tricky part of this last conversion, T4 to T3, is for those of you who are adrenal fatigued. When the adrenals are malfunctioning and cortisol levels are elevated, instead of making T3 you will make reverse T3, which is not a bioactive version of T3 and is of no use to your cells.

Knowing all that, now let's look at how fasting can help. We know that autophagy fasting repairs neurons in the brain, which is essential for TSH production and for your brain to receive hormonal communication from your body. We also know that fasting for 24 hours can help heal your gut, which is essential for conversion of T4 into T3. All fasts and keeping your glucose levels on the lower side force your body to release stored sugar from your liver, again making the conversion from T4 to T3 easier. All fasts also lower cellular inflammation, making it easier for T3 to get into the cells. Can you see how helpful fasting is to your thyroid function and the utilization of thyroid hormones?

One of the misconceptions I have heard over the years is that fasting lowers your thyroid hormones. I dove into the studies on that claim. In fact, I have done videos, interviewed thyroid experts on my podcast, and may be mildly obsessed with understanding fasting and thyroid function. Here is what the research shows: There is a temporary reduction in T3 when you fast, but there is some nuance here that you need to know. A study published in *Metabolism* showed that the effects were only temporary. Once food was put back in the subjects' diets, T3 levels shot up and, in some cases, were even higher than before.[1]

Fasting with adrenal fatigue

The key to succeeding at fasting with adrenal fatigue is to slowly back into your fasting lifestyle. Make small changes to your fasting window, growing it little by little over weeks, maybe months. Remember, a small amount of hormetic stress can help repair your adrenals. It's okay to gently push those adrenals, just not too much.

The other key to supporting your adrenals through a fasting experience is to be sure you stabilize your blood sugar with lots of good, healthy fats. If your blood sugar is more stable, not swinging from extreme highs to extreme lows, it will make it easier on your adrenals to fast. Lastly, there is more to adrenal fatigue than just the adrenals not doing their job. If you know that your adrenals are not at their best, reach out to a functional practitioner who can support you through your fasting process.

Fasting and pregnancy

Definitely do not fast when pregnant, for two reasons. First, you need to fuel and nourish both yourself and your baby. Food is your medicine at this moment, not fasting. You can lean in to foods that enhance your gut microbiome and pass your gut microbiome on to your baby. Second, you don't want to stimulate any detox reactions while you're pregnant. When you detox while you are fasting, the toxins will be released into the bloodstream and go into your baby. This is definitely not a healing response you are looking for.

Fasting and nursing

The same detox rule applies here: You don't want lots of detoxing going on while you're nursing, because toxins will go into your breast milk. Sometimes shorter fasts like intermittent fasting for 13 hours can be good, but nothing longer than that. You also want to collaborate with your doctor when making this decision.

Fasting and diabetes

Both type 1 and type 2 diabetics can thrive with fasting. But I do recommend working with a health practitioner if your condition is severe. I have seen some crazy miracles happen for diabetics with fasting, but again, I want you to be safe, so please make sure that you monitor your blood sugar numbers and do so under supervision. If your doctor is unfamiliar with fasting, point him or her to the meta-analysis on intermittent fasting published in *The New England Journal of Medicine* (noted in Chapter 2). Often doctors are not up to speed on what the current research is saying about fasting, and this peer-reviewed article can be extremely helpful for your doctor to read.

Fasting and eating disorders

Let me state strongly that if you have an eating disorder you need to involve your doctor in the process of building a fasting lifestyle. First and foremost, I want you to be safe. If you have a history of eating disorders, you also will need to work with your doctor to build your fasting lifestyle safely. There are several warning signs that will tell you that your fasting lifestyle is taking you down a dangerous mental path. The first is if you start focusing on restricting calories. Fasting is not about calorie restriction. Once you open up your eating window, please make sure you are eating enough high-quality food. The second is if you're looking at fasting as an excuse to start skipping meals. This is where you want your practitioner involved. Fasting is a therapeutic tool that can accelerate healing in your body, but you want to be strategic about how long you fast and which meals you skip. Third, if you start shaming yourself about breaking your fast too early or feel like you are failing, it might be time to back off on your fasting lifestyle. There is no such thing as a failed fast. This should feel like a compassionate journey that leads you to a mentally healthier place, not a rigid process you have to muscle your way through. If fasting can't be a positive experience, then I highly recommend you stop.

No doubt you will have more questions crop up as you fast. If these hacks don't help, I encourage you to find my online community, like my free Facebook group, the Resetter Collaborative. I also have published several hundred videos about fasting on my YouTube channel, many of them answering questions like the ones above. I am sure if you have questions that I haven't answered above, you will find them there!

CHAPTER 11

Recipes

Fasting like a girl doesn't mean you deprive your taste buds. Pairing your fasts with yummy foods will not only make your fasting lifestyle more fun, but it will help you effortlessly integrate these healing principles into your life long term. Below are some amazing recipes that will excite both your taste buds and your hormones. Be adventurous with these recipes. Don't shy away from a recipe that has a food you don't normally eat. Remember, a diversity of food choices only enhances your health. Enjoy!

Please note: Recipes with a (V) indicate a vegetarian selection.

KETOBIOTIC RECIPES

LOADED HUMMUS BOWL (V)

Makes 4 servings (1½ cups per serving)

Ingredients

Hummus

4 garlic cloves, divided
1 large lemon, juiced
One 14.5-ounce can chickpeas, drained and rinsed
½ teaspoon baking soda
⅓ cup tahini
Sea salt

Tempeh and greens

2 tablespoons olive oil
12 ounces tempeh, crumbled
1 teaspoon sea salt
1 teaspoon freshly ground black pepper
1 teaspoon cumin
½ teaspoon coriander
½ teaspoon cayenne pepper
4 cups spinach or baby kale

Toppings

½ cup pitted Castelvetrano olives, chopped
½ red onion, diced
1 cup cherry tomatoes, halved
¼ cup roasted pumpkin seeds
Extra-virgin olive oil

Sumac, cumin, or paprika

Instructions

Crush 2 of the garlic cloves with the flat side of your knife. Place them in a small bowl and cover them with the lemon juice. Set aside so the raw garlic can begin to mellow out in the acidic juice while you cook the chickpeas.

Combine the chickpeas, ½ teaspoon baking soda, and the remaining 2 garlic cloves in a large saucepan. Cover with water and bring to a boil over high heat. Once the mixture begins to boil, turn the heat down to medium and continue to boil gently for 25 to 30 minutes, or until the chickpeas are so tender that their skins are starting to fall off.

Strain the cooked chickpeas and garlic and transfer to a food processor. Add in the garlic with the lemon juice and tahini. Blend until smooth, and then slowly stream some filtered water into the food processor while it's running, adding just enough to help turn the texture from slightly grainy to a perfect velvety consistency. (This shouldn't take more than a couple of tablespoons.) Add the sea salt to taste, then set aside and prepare the tempeh and greens.

Heat the olive oil in a large skillet over medium-high heat. Add the crumbled tempeh and the next 5 ingredients. Stir and cook for a few minutes until the tempeh begins to turn golden and crisp at the edges, then add in the greens. Cook for another 1 to 2 minutes, just until the greens are slightly wilted.

Divide the hummus among 4 bowls, using the back of a spoon to create an even, wavy layer. Divide the tempeh and greens equally among the bowls, then top each serving with the olives, onions, tomatoes, and pumpkin seeds. Finish each bowl with a slight drizzle of olive oil and a dusting of sumac.

Nutritional Information

Per serving
Total Fat 31g
Net Carbohydrate 24g
Protein 28g

SHAVED BRUSSELS SPROUT SALAD WITH CHICKEN AND GINGER MISO DRESSING

Makes 4 servings (1½ cups per serving)

Ingredients

Chicken

2 boneless, skinless chicken breasts, halved
1 teaspoon sea salt
1 teaspoon freshly ground black pepper
1 teaspoon garlic powder
½ teaspoon onion powder
2 tablespoons avocado oil

Salad

4 cups brussels sprouts, trimmed and shaved
4 scallions, roots trimmed, sliced thin
¼ cup slivered almonds
2 tablespoons whole flaxseeds
2 tablespoons toasted sesame seeds

Dressing

¼ cup avocado oil

1 tablespoon toasted sesame oil
3 tablespoons rice vinegar
3 tablespoons coconut aminos
1 tablespoon freshly grated ginger
2 teaspoons white miso paste
1 garlic clove, grated

Instructions

Season all sides of the chicken with salt, pepper, garlic powder, and onion powder. Heat the avocado oil in a large skillet over medium-high heat. Add the chicken to the heated oil and cook for 5 to 6 minutes per side, or until golden and cooked through. Remove from the heat and set aside.

Toss together all the ingredients for the salad in a large bowl.

Place all the ingredients for the dressing in a medium bowl and whisk until fully combined.

Cut the chicken into bite-size pieces and add to the bowl of brussels sprout salad. Add the dressing, toss, and serve.

Nutritional Information

Per serving
Total Fat 15g
Net Carbohydrate 8g
Protein 28g

SHAKSHUKA WITH PICKLED ONIONS AND AVOCADO

Makes 4 servings (about 1½ cups per serving)

Ingredients

2 tablespoons olive oil
1 yellow onion, peeled and diced
4 garlic cloves, minced
1 red bell pepper, seeded and diced
3 tablespoons tomato paste
2 tablespoons harissa
1 teaspoon sea salt
1 teaspoon freshly ground black pepper
1 teaspoon cumin
½ teaspoon paprika
One 28-ounce can crushed tomatoes
2 cups baby kale
8 eggs
1 large avocado, pitted, scooped out of the skin, and sliced
1 cup pickled red onion
¼ cup chopped cilantro

Instructions

Place the olive oil in a large skillet over medium-high heat. Add the onion and cook for about 2 minutes, or until it starts to become translucent, then add in the garlic and bell pepper. Cook for another 2 minutes, then stir in the tomato paste, harissa, salt, pepper, cumin, and paprika. Stir and cook until the mixture becomes fragrant.

Stir in the crushed tomatoes, and if the sauce starts to boil or sputter, turn the heat down to a lower setting. Let the mixture simmer for 20 minutes (it will thicken slightly).

Add in the kale and cook until it wilts. Gently add in the eggs, one at a time, keeping the yolks intact. Cover the pan and cook for another 5 to 6 minutes, or until the eggs are set and the yolks are cooked to your preferred doneness.

Serve the shakshuka topped with the avocado, pickled onion, and cilantro.

Nutritional Information

Per serving
Total Fat 42g
Net Carbohydrate 27g
Protein 25g

KIMCHI SALAD WITH CRISPY CHICKPEAS (V)

Makes 4 servings (2 cups per serving)

Ingredients

Chickpeas

2 tablespoons olive oil
One 14.5-ounce can chickpeas, drained and rinsed
½ teaspoon sea salt
½ teaspoon garlic powder
½ teaspoon onion powder
½ teaspoon turmeric
½ teaspoon cumin

Dressing

¼ cup avocado oil
3 tablespoons rice vinegar
3 tablespoons coconut aminos
1 garlic clove, grated
Sea salt
Freshly ground black pepper

Salad

1 cup kimchi, drained and chopped
1 head of romaine lettuce, trimmed and chopped
2 cups baby spinach
8 radishes, trimmed and thinly sliced
2 tablespoons hemp seeds
2 tablespoons sesame seeds

Instructions

Heat the olive oil in a large skillet over medium-high heat. Add the chickpeas to the skillet.

Combine the salt, garlic powder, onion powder, turmeric, and cumin in a small bowl. Sprinkle the spice mixture over the chickpeas. Stir to distribute the spices evenly and cook until the chickpeas start to become golden and crispy along the edges. Remove from the heat and set aside.

Combine the avocado oil, vinegar, coconut aminos, and garlic in a small bowl. Whisk together and season the dressing with salt and pepper to taste.

Toss the salad components together in a large bowl. Scatter the crispy chickpeas on top of the salad, drizzle with the dressing, then toss and serve.

Nutritional Information

Per serving
Total Fat 47g
Cholesterol 0mg
Net Carbohydrate 20g
Protein 27g

ALMOND CHICKEN TENDERS AND SAUERKRAUT SLAW

Makes 4 servings (3 chicken tenders over ½ cup sauerkraut per serving)

Ingredients

Slaw

2 cups sauerkraut, drained
2 celery stalks, thinly sliced
1 large Granny Smith apple, cored, halved, and thinly sliced
¼ cup apple cider vinegar
¼ cup roasted pumpkin seeds, hemp seeds, or flaxseeds
2 tablespoons avocado oil

Chicken

½ cup almond meal
3 tablespoons nutritional yeast
1½ teaspoons sea salt
1 teaspoon freshly ground black pepper
1 teaspoon paprika
1 teaspoon garlic powder
½ teaspoon onion powder
1 egg
½ cup unsweetened almond milk
1 pound chicken tenderloins
2 tablespoons avocado oil

Instructions

Preheat the oven to 400°F.

Line a baking sheet with parchment paper and set aside.

Combine all the ingredients for the slaw in a large bowl and toss to combine. Season with salt to taste, if desired, then cover and place in the refrigerator while you make the tenders.

Combine the almond meal, yeast, salt, pepper, paprika, garlic powder, and onion powder in a large shallow bowl or pie plate.

Whisk together the egg and almond milk in a separate wide-brimmed bowl.

Set up a dredging station. Start by dipping both sides of a chicken tender into the egg mixture, then gently press and roll the chicken in the almond meal coating. Place the chicken on the prepared baking sheet once it's fully coated. Repeat until all the tenders are coated. Gently brush the oil over the top of the tenderloins. Place in the oven and bake for 35 to 40 minutes.

Serve the chicken tenders with a helping of the slaw.

Nutritional Information

Per serving
Total Fat 35g
Cholesterol 148mg
Net Carbohydrate 13g
Protein 49g

GARLIC-GINGER TEMPEH AND BROCCOLI OVER QUINOA (V)

Makes 4 servings (about 2 cups per serving)

Ingredients

6 garlic cloves, minced
2 tablespoons freshly grated ginger
2 tablespoons toasted sesame oil
⅓ cup coconut aminos
1 large lemon, juiced and zested
2 tablespoons avocado oil
12 ounces tempeh, cut into thin strips or crumbled
2 cups broccoli florets
Sea salt
Freshly ground pepper
1 cup quinoa, prepared according to the package instructions
1½ cups kimchi

Instructions

Combine the first 5 ingredients in a medium bowl. Whisk together and set aside.

Heat the oil in a large skillet over medium-high heat. Add the tempeh, cooking until the edges begin to turn golden brown, then add the broccoli. Season with salt and pepper to taste and cook for about 4 minutes. Reduce heat to medium and pour in the garlic-ginger mixture.

Cook until the sauce thickens and the broccoli is fork tender. Serve over the prepared quinoa with a side of kimchi.

Nutritional Information

Per serving
Total Fat 31g
Cholesterol 0mg
Net Carbohydrate 35g
Protein 40g

KIMCHI STEW WITH TOFU (V)

Makes 4 servings (about 1½ cups per serving)

Ingredients

2 tablespoons avocado oil
1 yellow onion, diced
6 garlic cloves, minced
3 cups kimchi, chopped
2 tablespoons chili paste
5 cups vegetable broth
1 15 ounce can cannellini or navy beans, drained and rinsed
Sea salt
Freshly ground black pepper
12 ounces extra-firm tofu, cubed
4 scallions, thinly sliced
¼ cup cilantro, chopped
Toasted sesame oil

Instructions

Heat the avocado oil in a large pot over medium-high heat. Add the onion and garlic and cook for 2 to 3 minutes, or until the onion starts to become translucent.

Add in the kimchi and chili paste. Stir and cook for 1 minute, then pour in the broth, add the beans, and season with salt and pepper to taste. Once the mixture begins to boil, reduce the heat to medium-low, then cover and simmer for 20 minutes.

Add the tofu to the pot, cover, and cook for another 15 minutes. If the stew is boiling before you add the tofu, turn down the heat to a simmer.

Serve the stew with the scallions, cilantro, and a drizzle of toasted sesame oil on top.

Nutritional Information

Per serving
Total Fat 22g
Net Carbohydrate 20g
Protein 41g

PROSCIUTTO, SPINACH, AND ASPARAGUS FRITTATA

Makes 8 servings (1 slice per serving)

Ingredients

8 eggs
½ cup unsweetened almond milk
⅓ cup nutritional yeast
1 teaspoon sea salt
1 teaspoon freshly ground black pepper
2 tablespoons ghee
1 large shallot, finely diced
3 garlic cloves, minced
4 ounces prosciutto, chopped
1 pound asparagus, woody ends removed, cut into 2- to 3-inch pieces
3 cups spinach

Instructions

Preheat the oven to 350°F.

Heat a large cast-iron pan (or other oven-safe pan) over medium-high heat.

Combine the eggs, almond milk, yeast, salt, and pepper in a medium bowl. Whisk thoroughly and set aside.

Add in the ghee once the pan becomes hot.

Wait for the ghee to melt, then add in the shallot and garlic. Cook for 1 to 2 minutes, or until the shallot starts to become translucent, then add in the prosciutto. Cook for another 3 to 4 minutes. Add the asparagus once the prosciutto starts to become golden and crispy.

Cook until the asparagus becomes bright green, then add in the spinach and cook for a couple of minutes, or until the spinach wilts.

Pour the egg mixture over the sautéed vegetables. Cook for 3 to 4 minutes, or just until the bottom of the frittata begins to set. Transfer the frittata to the oven and bake for 15 minutes, or until the eggs are cooked through at the center.

Cut the frittata like a pie and serve.

Nutritional Information

Per serving
Total Fat 20g
Net Carbohydrate 8g
Protein 33g

BRATS WITH SAUTÉED APPLES AND ONIONS (SERVE WITH SAUERKRAUT)

Makes 4 servings (1½ cups per serving)

Ingredients

2 tablespoons olive oil
1 pound brats, cut into medallions
1 large onion, halved and thinly sliced
2 Granny Smith apples, cored, peeled, and thinly sliced
¼ cup apple cider vinegar
¼ cup seeds such as flax, pumpkin, hemp, or a combo of all 3
1 teaspoon smoked paprika
Sea salt
Freshly ground black pepper
1½ cups sauerkraut

Instructions

Heat the olive oil in a large skillet over medium-high heat. Add the brats, stirring to sear evenly, and cook for about 2 minutes. Add in the onion.

Continue cooking for 5 to 6 minutes, or until the onion becomes soft and translucent (close to caramelized). Add in the apples, vinegar, seeds, and paprika and season with salt and pepper to taste.

Cook for another few minutes, or until the apples are tender and the liquid has reduced by more than half.

Serve with a scoop of sauerkraut.

Nutritional Information

Per serving
Total Fat 55g
Net Carbohydrate 20g

Protein 26g

COCONUT AND KALE LENTIL SOUP (V)

Makes 4 servings (1½ cups per serving)

Ingredients

1 cup unsweetened shredded coconut
2 tablespoons avocado oil
1 yellow onion, diced
6 garlic cloves, minced
2 tablespoons freshly grated ginger
2 tablespoons red curry paste
1 cup red split lentils
5 cups vegetable broth
1 teaspoon salt
1 teaspoon freshly ground black pepper
One 14.5-ounce can full-fat coconut milk
4 cups kale, stems removed, chopped
¼ cup seeds of your choosing (pumpkin, flax, hemp)

Instructions

Heat a large pot over medium-high heat. Once the pot is hot, add the shredded coconut. Dry toast the coconut in the pot, stirring continuously, until it starts to turn a light golden brown. Immediately transfer the toasted coconut to a medium bowl and set aside.

Return the pot to the stove and add the avocado oil. Add the onion and cook for 2 to 3 minutes, or until it just starts to become translucent, then add in the garlic and ginger. Stir and cook for less than a minute, then add in the red curry paste.

Continue to stir over the heat until the mixture becomes fragrant.

Add in the lentils, broth, salt, pepper, and the reserved toasted coconut. Once the mixture boils, reduce the heat to medium-low, cover, and simmer for 25 to 30 minutes, or until the lentils are tender and cooked through.

Stir in the coconut milk and kale a few minutes before serving. Keep the soup over the heat until the kale wilts. Season the soup with more salt and pepper to taste and serve with a sprinkle of seeds on top.

Nutritional Information

Per serving
Total Fat 40g
Net Carbohydrate 24g
Protein 21g

PULLED PORK IN BONE BROTH

Makes 12 servings (1 cup per serving)

Ingredients

1 teaspoon salt (or to taste)
½ teaspoon pepper (or to taste)
6 pounds pork shoulder
8 cups Basic Beef Bone Broth
Juice of 2 lemons
2 tablespoons ground cumin
3 to 4 bay leaves
2 tablespoons ground herbes de Provence

½ teaspoon cayenne pepper
¼ cup chopped cilantro
1 medium organic yellow onion, cored
1 teaspoon arrowroot powder

Instructions

Braising can be done in 4 ways. Here are the fastest to slowest methods: pressure cooker (1 hour), stovetop (3 to 4 hours), oven (4 to 8 hours), or slow cooker (also 4 to 8 hours). The slow cooker method is the least time intensive; it should hold 6-plus quarts (that's what these directions are for).

Sprinkle salt and pepper over the entire pork shoulder. Heat a large frying or sauté pan on medium-high heat. Place the meat in the pan and sear each side to a light golden brown. This is an important step because you're doing 2 things that are going to make your final dish delicious: sealing in moisture and creating flavor. All the crusty bits are full of flavor that will transfer to your braising liquid.

Boil the Basic Beef Bone Broth and lemon juice with the spices before putting the mixture into the slow cooker.

Put the liquids, meat, and onion into the slow cooker and cook on low for 8 hours. Note that the liquid should just cover the meat.

When you're finished cooking, you can set aside some of the Basic Beef Bone Broth to mix in with the shredded meat, but first you'll want to thicken it a little bit with some arrowroot powder. This is done by mixing a little hot liquid with a teaspoon of arrowroot powder at a time, thoroughly blending, then adding it back to your reserved liquid for sauce.

Remove the meat from the slow cooker and shred, using 2 forks, and add the thickened sauce.

Nutritional Information

Per serving
Total Fat 3g
Net Carbohydrate 1g
Protein 25g

BACON-AVO-EGG (BACON, AVOCADO, EGG)

Makes 4 servings (1 avocado per serving)

Ingredients

4 large avocados
1 teaspoon salt
¼ cup raw apple cider vinegar
4 large free-range chicken or duck eggs
16 slices hormone-free bacon

Instructions

Halve the avocados and discard the seeds. Scoop a small amount of avocado out of the center to make room for the poached egg that will go inside. Carefully peel off the avocado skin. Set aside.

Fill a saucepan with 3 to 4 inches of water. Add ½ teaspoon of salt and the apple cider vinegar and bring to a boil. Poach eggs for 5 minutes.

Carefully place 1 poached egg into one half of an avocado and close it inside by covering with the other half. Wrap each avocado with approximately 4 slices of bacon.

Set a curved pan over high heat. Sear the bacon on the outside of the avocado, rotating it slowly until it's crispy and golden brown all around. Leaning the avocado along the edge of a curved pan is a great way to sear the curved areas. Once the bacon starts to cook and get crisp, it will create a shell and hold the avocado together and the egg inside.

Serve immediately.

Tips and tricks:

The acid in the water from the vinegar is what helps keep the egg together while poaching. The trick to searing the bacon-wrapped avocado is high heat: It has to be hot and fast; otherwise, the texture of the soft avocado underneath will be compromised. Serve this delicious dish over a salad of mixed greens, sliced heirloom tomatoes, freshly chopped parsley, and crumbled feta cheese.

Nutritional Information

Per serving
Total Fat 59g
Net Carbohydrate 9g
Protein 117g

ROASTED LEG OF LAMB

Makes 20 servings (4 ounces per serving)

Ingredients

5 pounds boneless leg of lamb
8 fresh rosemary sprigs
Zest and juice of 2 lemons
1 tablespoon minced garlic
¼ cup avocado oil
2 teaspoons salt
1 teaspoon ground pepper
Two 10-gallon clear plastic garbage bags

Instructions

Place all the ingredients into 2 (for extra strength) 10-gallon clear plastic garbage bags. Take extra care when adding the rosemary sprigs to make sure they don't puncture the plastic. Get all the air out of the bags and tie a knot at the top; this makes sure that the entire leg of lamb gets marinated.

Place the lamb in a bowl or on a dish (just in case it leaks) and set in the fridge to marinate for 4 hours or up to 2 days.

Cook the lamb on the grill over medium heat for 45 minutes, or until cooked through. Or start it on the grill to get color and then finish it in the oven set at 375°F for 45 minutes or until done.

Nutritional Information

Per serving
Total Fat 17g
Net Carbohydrate 0g
Protein 21g

THE BEST ROASTED CHICKEN

Makes 4 servings (4 ounces per serving)

Ingredients

1 whole chicken
3 lemons, sliced
5 fresh rosemary sprigs
1 teaspoon sea salt
½ teaspoon ground pepper
Dash of paprika

Instructions

Preheat the oven to 375°F.

Prepare a roasting pan by covering it with parchment paper and tucking the edges between the drip pan.

Butterfly your chicken by removing the spine. You can do this either with sturdy kitchen shears or with a knife. By removing the spine, you can flatten the chicken out on the roasting pan so that it cooks more evenly and in less time, all the while staying moist on the inside and crispy on the outside.

Create a bed of lemon slices and rosemary sprigs in the bottom of the parchment-lined roasting pan.

Place the chicken on top of the lemons and rosemary. Sprinkle with the salt, pepper, and paprika.

Roast the chicken for 45 to 55 minutes, or until the juices run clear.

Nutritional Information

Per serving

Total Fat 6g
Net Carbohydrate 0g
Protein 25g

KETOBIOTIC WAFFLES

Makes 16 waffles (2 waffles per serving)

Ingredients

3 cups blanched almond flour
¼ cup shredded coconut, unsweetened
1 teaspoon baking powder
¼ teaspoon sea salt
½ teaspoon ground cinnamon
⅔ cup coconut milk
¼ cup maple syrup
2 teaspoons vanilla extract
5 free-range eggs, yolks and whites separated
⅓ cup grass-fed butter, softened

For chocolate waffles, add ¼ cup raw cacao powder.

Instructions

Turn on your waffle iron to the desired setting.

Combine all the dry ingredients in a medium bowl and stir until evenly mixed.

Cream the coconut milk, maple syrup, vanilla, egg yolks, and butter in a large bowl.

Beat the egg whites to a soft peak in a separate medium bowl.

Gently fold the egg whites into the egg-yolk mixture in the large bowl.

Gently fold the dry ingredients into the creamed liquid ingredients until fully incorporated.

Using a 2-ounce ladle, position a dollop of batter onto the center of the waffle square. Cook per the waffle iron instructions (approximately 4 minutes). Continue cooking until all the waffle batter is used.

Nutritional Information

Per serving
Total Fat 23g
Net Carbohydrate 3g
Protein 5g

CRUSTLESS EVERYTHING QUICHE

Makes 8 servings (1 slice per serving)

Ingredients

1 cup diced onion, sautéed until clear
3 cups (total) of whatever you have in your kitchen, such as:
1 cup frozen organic spinach, thawed, squeezed, finely diced
1 cup diced bacon, cooked
1 cup diced (½-inch cubes) butternut squash
1 cup diced roasted red bell peppers
3 cups (total) of whatever cheese you have, such as:
1½ cups shredded goat cheddar cheese
1½ cups shredded raw Parmesan cheese
8 large free-range eggs, beaten

½ teaspoon salt
½ teaspoon pepper
1 teaspoon of the herb of your choice (mine is herbes de Provence)

Instructions

Preheat the oven to 350°F.

Lightly grease an 8-inch square baking dish with butter.

Prep your ingredients: Sauté the onion. Thaw, squeeze, and chop the spinach. Cook and chop the bacon. Dice the roasted bell pepper. Grate the cheeses.

Beat the eggs, then add the salt, pepper, and spices.

Mix all the ingredients together in a large bowl.

Pour the mixture into the greased baking dish. Bake for 30 to 40 minutes, or until a toothpick inserted in the center comes out clean.

Tips and tricks:

As long as you keep the proportions the same in this recipe, you can experiment with different ingredients. This quiche never gets boring!

Nutritional Information

Per serving
Total Fat 20g
Net Carbohydrate 15g
Protein 11g

BREADCRUMB-FREE CRAB CAKES

Makes 6 crab cakes (1 crab cake per serving)

Ingredients

½ head of cauliflower, riced, steamed, and water extracted (1 cup when finished)
5 free-range eggs
3 tablespoons Garlic Avocado Aioli (Store-bought is fine)
¼ cup finely chopped curly parsley
½ teaspoon sea salt
¼ teaspoon ground pepper
½ teaspoon cayenne pepper
½ teaspoon paprika
1 teaspoon fresh dill
6 tablespoons coconut flour
1 pound responsibly sourced crabmeat, cooked
2 tablespoons avocado oil or coconut oil (for searing)
Lemon juice to taste

Instructions

Rice the cauliflower in a powerful blender or food processor. Steam for 10 minutes. Squeeze out the excess liquid, either with cheesecloth, a kitchen towel, or a nut milk bag. Set aside to cool.

Whisk together the eggs, Garlic Avocado Aioli, and spices in a small bowl.

Gently fold the cold cauliflower with the egg mixture and coconut flour in a medium bowl until evenly mixed. (It's important that the cauliflower is cold so that it won't cook the eggs.) The cauliflower and the coconut flour give the finished crab cakes a nice, crispy outside.

Gently fold in the crabmeat, being careful not to break up the meat too much. (It's nice when the finished crab cakes have large chunks of meat in them.)

Cool the mixture in the fridge for 15 minutes, and preheat the oven to 350°F.

Make the patties, approximately 1 inch thick and 3 inches across.

Pour the oil into a cast-iron (recommended) pan set over medium-high heat. When the pan and oil are hot, add the crab cakes, being careful not to overcrowd the pan (this will cause steaming, not searing). Cook the crab cakes for about 3 minutes to a golden brown, then flip over and cook another 3 minutes.

Transfer the pan-fried crab cakes to a baking sheet and place in the oven to cook through, about 12 to 15 minutes. Squeeze the lemons over the patties to taste.

Tips and tricks:

Serve over mixed greens with half an avocado.

Nutritional Information

Per serving
Total Fat 4g
Net Carbohydrate 2g
Protein 10g

HEALTHY CHICKEN NUGGETS

Makes 48 chicken nuggets (6 nuggets per serving)

Ingredients

8 boneless, skinless free-range hormone-free chicken breasts
3 cups quinoa flour
2 teaspoons garlic powder
2 teaspoons sea salt
2 teaspoons ground black pepper
4 eggs, beaten
1 cup coconut oil

Instructions

Cut the chicken into nugget-shaped pieces (about 6 nuggets per chicken breast).

Mix the flour, garlic powder, salt, and pepper thoroughly in a shallow dish. Dip the chicken pieces individually into the beaten eggs, then coat each side lightly with the flour mixture. Shake off any excess flour before placing on a plate; continue until all the chicken has been coated.

Liberally coat a large nonreactive skillet or saucepan (cast iron is my favorite) with coconut oil. You want to use enough so that the chicken nuggets don't have dry spots but not so much that they're soggy.

Sauté the nuggets for 4 minutes on each side until golden brown. You may need to pause between batches to quickly clean the pan of any small bits that remain; those tend to burn if not removed, making the conditions less than ideal for the fresh nuggets.

You'll know that your nuggets are done when they're golden brown and no longer pink in the center. This will be about 12 minutes per batch.

Nutritional Information

Per serving
Total Fat 29g
Net Carbohydrate 3g
Protein 48g

PURPLE GOLD KRAUT (V)

Makes 14 cups (1 cup per serving)

Ingredients

2 heads of organic red cabbage, shredded
⅓ cup fresh organic turmeric, finely grated
⅓ cup fresh organic ginger, finely grated
2 tablespoons sea salt
2 tablespoons apple cider vinegar

Additional brine

4 cups purified water
4 teaspoons sea salt
4 teaspoons apple cider vinegar

Instructions

Pull 4 to 5 large leaves off of 1 of the heads of cabbage and set aside. Shred the remaining cabbage.

Mix the shredded cabbage, turmeric, ginger, salt, and vinegar in a large bowl. (Use a stainless steel bowl because the turmeric won't stain it bright yellow.) Wearing gloves to keep your hands from getting stained, massage the cabbage mixture with your hands until it breaks down and starts to soften, about 5 to 10 minutes. Let the mixture sit for 20 to 30 minutes to give it time to continue to macerate and release more juices.

Massage the mixture for another 5 to 10 minutes.

Pack the cabbage mixture into two 36-ounce mason jars with a large, long-handled spoon. Pack the mixture in tightly, all the way down to the bottom. You want the mixture to be submerged in brine (the natural juices created through the maceration process). Leave about 1½ inches of space from the top of the jar.

Typically you will need to make additional brine. This is done by combining water with the sea salt and apple cider vinegar. Continue to add brine until the cabbage mixture is submerged.

Roll up the cabbage leaves you set aside and place them in the jar to push the cabbage under the brine. Screw the jar lid on loosely so gas can escape as fermentation takes place. Set on the counter for 5 to 14 days in a cool, shaded place. During fermentation, the sauerkraut will bubble a little and become cloudy. If scum or mold appears at the top or on the whole cabbage leaves, remove and discard; replace with new cabbage leaves to keep the cabbage submerged.

Taste the sauerkraut every day. When you like the flavor, remove the rolled-up cabbage leaves and place the sauerkraut in the refrigerator, which slows down the fermentation process.

Tips and tricks:

Wear gloves and clothes that can get stained when making this recipe; the turmeric juice will stain your hands and could permanently stain your clothes. Fruit such as pineapple can accelerate the fermentation process and might take less time to achieve a flavor of your liking. After 5 to 6 days, the sauerkraut is crunchy and deliciously fresh. After about 10 days, the flavor gets a little tarter and the texture is softer. This sauerkraut is the perfect accompaniment for a break-fast dish.

Nutritional Information

Per serving
Total Fat 0g
Net Carbohydrate 2g
Protein 0g

YELLOW CAULIFLOWER TORTILLAS

Makes 12 tortillas (2 tortillas per serving)

Ingredients

2 heads of cauliflower, steamed (yields approximately 8 cups chopped cauliflower)
1 cup chopped green onions (approximately 2 bunches)
5 large free-range eggs, beaten
½ teaspoon sea salt
½ teaspoon finely ground black pepper
½ teaspoon ground turmeric
¾ teaspoon xanthan gum

Instructions

Preheat the oven to 350°F.

Steam the cauliflower heads until tender, about 4 to 5 minutes. Blend the cauliflower and green onions in a food processor or powerful blender until smooth (they will have a slightly green color because of the onions; don't worry, once you add the turmeric, they'll turn yellow). This mixture should make about 32 fluid ounces.

Strain the mixture through cheesecloth or a nut milk bag to get rid of any excess liquid.

Mix together the cauliflower mixture, eggs, salt, pepper, turmeric, and xanthan gum in a medium bowl.

Pour ¼ cup of batter for each tortilla onto a baking sheet lined with parchment paper or a nonstick silicone baking liner.

Bake for 25 minutes on 1 side only.

Let cool before removing from the baking sheet.

Tips and tricks:

These tortillas can be made in advance and stored in the fridge for a few days; make sure you layer them in between parchment paper.

Nutritional Information

Per serving
Total Fat 1g
Net Carbohydrate 22g
Protein 3g

FRESH MINT AND PEA SPREAD

Makes 3 cups (24 servings, 2 tablespoons per serving)

Ingredients

3 cups fresh English peas
½ cup almonds, ground to consistency of flour
Zest of 1 lemon
2 cups fresh mint, well packed
3 tablespoons lemon juice
1 shishito pepper
2 ounces goat cheese
½ cup avocado oil

Instructions

Place all the ingredients into a powerful blender and blend on medium speed until the spread is the desired consistency.

Store in the refrigerator in a glass container. The spread will last in the fridge for 5 to 7 days.

Nutritional Information

Per serving
Total Fat 0g
Net Carbohydrate 8g
Protein 4g

MEYER LEMON–GINGER SALMON

Makes 12 servings (4 ounces per serving)

Ingredients

1 to 2 tablespoons sesame oil
1 large wild salmon fillet (2½ to 3 pounds)
2 tablespoons low-sodium organic miso
1 tablespoon coconut aminos

4 tablespoons grated fresh ginger
½ teaspoon grated fresh turmeric
2 teaspoons minced garlic
2 teaspoons raw local honey
Juice from 2 large Meyer lemons
Zest from 3 large Meyer lemons

Instructions

Preheat the oven to 350°F.

Prepare a large baking dish (15 inches is a perfect size) by adding a little sesame oil to the bottom of the pan before you lay in the salmon, skin-side down. (This will prevent the skin from sticking.)

Mix the remaining ingredients together in a small bowl, forming a thick sauce. Pack the sauce on top of the salmon. (The thick, zesty part of the sauce will stay on top and create a crust during the baking process, and the juices will slide to the bottom of the pan, giving flavor and moisture to the rest of the fish.)

Bake for approximately 45 minutes, or until the salmon starts to brown on the top and is cooked through in the thickest part of the fillet.

Tips and tricks:

If your fillet is too long for your baking dish, you can cut off the small tail end of the salmon and place it in the empty space in the baking dish; it does not have to be cooked in one piece. Watch the thinner areas of the salmon to make sure they don't overcook and get dry; if you need to, you can take these parts out early.

Nutritional Information

Per serving
Total Fat 42g
Net Carbohydrate 1g
Protein 50g

BRAISED BEEF COLLAGEN BOOST

Makes 24 servings (4 ounces per serving)

Ingredients

4 to 4½ cups beef bone broth (see recipe for Basic Beef Bone Broth)
8 pounds organic grass-fed beef
1 tablespoon sea salt for searing
1 tablespoon ground black pepper for searing
1 onion, peeled and cut into 8 wedges
12 ounces tomato paste (buy only brands that come in glass containers)
2 cups carrots (3 to 4 large carrots, cut into 2-inch chunks)
4 celery stalks, cut into 2-inch-long chunks
1 tablespoon ground herbes de Provence
4 to 5 whole garlic cloves

Instructions

You can braise 4 ways. Here are the fastest to slowest methods: pressure cooker, stovetop, oven, or slow cooker. These directions are for a 6-plus-quart slow cooker.

Start warming up the bone broth in your slow cooker. Sometimes, I boil the bone broth first to help kick-start it.

Prepare to sear your beef by sprinkling salt and pepper on all surfaces. Heat a large frying or sauté pan on medium-high heat and sear each side of the meat until lightly golden brown. This is an important step because you're doing 2 things that are going to make your final dish delicious: sealing in moisture and creating flavor. All the crusty bits are full of flavor that will transfer to your braising liquid.

Place the meat and all the remaining ingredients in the slow cooker. Braise for 4 to 8 hours. (I go the whole 8 hours so that the meat is as tender as possible and ready to eat when I'm finished with my workday.)

Tips and tricks:

Use a 6 ½-quart slow cooker in the A.M. Braised meats only get better the longer the flavors meld together, and it's like having a free meal that I didn't have to invest time in. This is why this recipe is made to feed a small army: Eat some, freeze some, give some away!

Before serving, you can choose to take some sauce to serve with your braised beef by transferring 1½ cups of the sauce to a saucepan. In a small glass, mix a small amount of warm liquid with 1 to 2 teaspoons of arrowroot powder; use a small whisk to blend. Then incorporate this mixture into the sauce you've set aside in the saucepan. This premixing technique minimizes clumping.

Nutritional Information

Per serving
Total Fat 13g
Net Carbohydrate 0g
Protein 13g

SALMON IN PARCHMENT PAPER

Makes 8 servings (2 ounces per serving)

Ingredients

16 ounces asparagus
2 yellow bell peppers, thinly sliced
1 red onion, thinly sliced
4 large tomatoes, diced
4 tablespoons capers, drained
8 salmon fillets
2 lemons, juiced
¼ cup avocado oil
3 lemons, sliced
1 teaspoon sea salt
1 teaspoon ground pepper
½ teaspoon cayenne pepper
½ cup basil, thinly sliced

Instructions

Preheat the oven to 400°F.

Cut parchment paper into eight 17-inch squares.

Divide asparagus, bell peppers, onion, tomatoes, and capers evenly among the 8 parchment squares. Place 1 salmon fillet on top of each. Drizzle lemon juice and a little avocado oil over each piece of salmon. Top with 1 to 2 lemon slices, salt, pepper, and a dash of cayenne. Bring the parchment paper sides up over the salmon; double-fold the top and sides to seal, making airtight pockets. Place the pockets on a baking sheet.

Bake the salmon for 15 to 20 minutes; your thermometer should register 140°F to 145°F when inserted through the paper and into the fish. Place each packet on a separate plate and cut open. Sprinkle some basil over the top of the fish and serve immediately.

Tips and tricks:

The parchment paper keeps the fish moist, as well as keeping all the flavor in! This dish is a winner with dinner guests, too, because it looks fancy when you serve it in the parchment paper.

Nutritional Information

Per serving
Total Fat 8g
Net Carbohydrate 1g
Protein 10g

YELLOWED CAULIFLOWER (V)

Makes 8 to 12 servings (1 cup per serving)

Ingredients

2 large heads of cauliflower
1½ teaspoons ground turmeric
1 teaspoon sea salt
½ teaspoon pepper
⅓ cup avocado oil
1 pair disposable plastic gloves (for prep)

Instructions

Preheat the oven to 350°F.

Remove the tough core from the cauliflower and break the rest into 3-inch florets.

Mix the turmeric, salt, and pepper in a small bowl and reserve.

Place the cauliflower in a large rectangular baking dish. Drizzle the avocado oil over the cauliflower and toss to coat evenly. (Use the gloves so your hands don't turn bright yellow!) Sprinkle the spices over the cauliflower and continue tossing to coat evenly.

Roast the cauliflower in the oven for 45 minutes, mixing and tossing twice during cooking time to ensure even cooking.

Enjoy the roasted cauliflower with steak, chicken, salmon, shrimp—almost anything!

Tips and tricks:

Any leftovers are great served cold on a salad!

Nutritional Information

Per serving
Total Fat 10g
Net Carbohydrate 3g
Protein 4g

GREEN BEANS WITH CARAMELIZED SHALLOTS

Makes 10 servings (1 cup per serving)

Ingredients

15 shallots

1 to 2 tablespoons avocado oil
2 pounds green beans
1 cup sliced almonds
2 tablespoons grass-fed butter
1 teaspoon salt
½ teaspoon pepper

Instructions

Prepare the shallots by peeling and slicing thinly. Place the shallots and 1 tablespoon of the avocado oil in a medium frying pan and sauté until the shallots are caramelized and golden brown (this may take 30 minutes—add more oil if necessary). Stir occasionally, but not too often; the shallots need time to cook, and if you stir too often, the caramelization doesn't have time to happen. But at the same time, keep a watchful eye on them so they don't burn. Once caramelized, reserve the shallots in a bowl.

Prepare to blanch the beans. Boil enough water to submerge the beans in an 8-quart stockpot. While the water is heating, trim both ends of the beans. Prepare an ice bath to cool the beans after blanching by adding ice and cold water to a large bowl. Boil the beans in the stockpot for about 3 minutes, then quickly transfer them to the ice bath to stop the cooking process. Once the beans are cool, remove them from the ice bath, drain, and reserve.

Lightly toast the sliced almonds in a frying pan over medium heat. The goal is to get the nuts just slightly brown to release the oils and produce an extra nutty flavor.

Five minutes before you're ready to serve, heat the butter in a large sauté or frying pan over medium-high heat. Add the green beans, salt, and pepper to the butter in the pan. Once the beans are hot, add in the caramelized shallots and sliced almonds. Mix evenly and serve.

Tips and tricks:

Blanching the beans for a short period of time and then reserving them until just before you're ready to serve will help you get them to the table hot and perfectly cooked.

Nutritional Information

Per serving
Total Fat 2g
Net Carbohydrate 7g
Protein 2g

CARDAMOM CARROT FRIES (V)

Makes 8 servings (1 cup per serving)

Ingredients

8 cups carrot sticks (start with 6 pounds large organic carrots)
2 tablespoons avocado oil
3 teaspoons ground herbes de Provence
1½ teaspoons chili powder
2 tablespoons cardamom (adjust to taste)
1/16 teaspoon cayenne pepper
1½ teaspoons salt
¼ teaspoon pepper

Instructions

Preheat the oven to 375°F.

Peel the carrots and start to prepare "fries" by cutting the carrots into even lengths. Then "square off" the carrots, eliminating the round edges. Once you have square columns of carrots, slice them into the thickness of your desired fries. Cut these slices into fries.

Place the carrot fries and the avocado oil in a large bowl and toss to coat evenly. Add the remaining ingredients and toss to incorporate evenly.

Line 2 large baking sheets with parchment paper or nonstick baking liners. Arrange the fries so they're not touching each other. You'll get the best results if each fry has space around it so that all can brown evenly.

Bake for 30 to 45 minutes, checking every 10 minutes or so to make sure they are cooking evenly.

Tips and tricks:

To get the traditional fries shape, you'll need to start with a lot of carrots, as eliminating the round parts reduces the number of finished carrots. You can have more fries if you're okay with a nontraditional shape. I like these carrot fries so much that I make four times the herb-salt-and-pepper mixture and store it in a spice jar to save a little time the next time I make these!

Nutritional Information

Per serving
Total Fat 14g
Net Carbohydrate 20g
Protein 3g

SPICY ZUCCHINI APPLE MUFFINS

Makes 24 muffins (1 muffin per serving)

Ingredients

2 cups grated zucchini
2 cups grated green apple
6 Medjool dates
1 cup nut butter
4 eggs
¼ cup coconut oil, melted
3 teaspoons vanilla extract
1 cup almond flour
1 teaspoon baking powder
½ teaspoon baking soda
4 teaspoons ground cinnamon
1 teaspoon ground ginger
1 teaspoon freshly ground nutmeg
¾ teaspoon allspice
¾ teaspoon ground cloves
½ teaspoon salt

Instructions

Preheat the oven to 350°F.

Grate the zucchini and apple with the peel on. Squeeze out the excess liquid from the zucchini.

Smash the dates, removing the pits, using a mortar and pestle or mince them in a food processor until they resemble a paste.

Blend the nut butter, eggs, and smashed dates in a large bowl. Mix in the zucchini, apple, coconut oil, and vanilla and blend thoroughly.

Place the remaining ingredients in a separate bowl and mix together. Incorporate the dry mixture into the wet mixture and blend evenly.

Lightly oil a silicone muffin pan or silicone muffin cups. If you don't have silicone, simply put paper liners in the muffin pan. Add about ¼ cup of batter to each cup.

Bake the muffins for 15 to 20 minutes, or until a toothpick comes out clean from the center.

Nutritional Information

Per serving
Total Fat 2g
Net Carbohydrate 20g
Protein 3g

ALMOND COCONUT BREAD

Makes 2 loaves (15 slices per loaf, 2 slices per serving)

Ingredients

2 cups almond flour
1½ cups coconut flour
⅔ cup hemp seeds
½ cup ground flaxseed
½ cup whole psyllium husks
2 tablespoons baking powder
2 teaspoons ground anise seed (optional, or spice of choice)
2 teaspoons salt
12 eggs, room temperature
1 cup raw cheddar cheese, grated

⅔ cup coconut oil, melted
1½ cups raw-milk kefir

Instructions

Preheat the oven to 350°F.

Combine all the dry ingredients in a large bowl. Stir well to incorporate the seeds evenly.

Beat the eggs in a separate large bowl, then incorporate the other wet ingredients until a smooth batter is formed.

Slowly incorporate the dry ingredients into the wet ingredients. (The coconut oil might clump a bit, but this will work itself out during baking.) Mix thoroughly. Pour the batter into two greased loaf pans lined with parchment paper.

Bake for 45 to 50 minutes, or until a toothpick inserted into the center comes out clean.

Remove from the oven, then remove the loaves from the pans and cool directly on a cooling rack so the crust dries; the bread will get soggy if it cools in the pan.

Let the loaves cool completely before slicing. Slice and toast right away, or slice and store in the freezer.

Nutritional Information

Per serving
Total Fat 10g
Net Carbohydrate 31g
Protein 3g

MINDY'S MAGIC SALAD DRESSING (V)

Makes 7 servings (2 ounces per serving)

Ingredients

¼ cup red wine vinegar
⅔ cup Meyer lemon juice
Zest of Meyer lemons
1 tablespoon raw honey
¾ cup olive oil
1½ teaspoons sea salt
1½ teaspoons ground pepper
¼ teaspoon cayenne pepper

Instructions

Blend all ingredients together.

Store in the refrigerator.

Shake before serving.

Tips and tricks:

This salad dressing tastes like summer all year long! Add some finely chopped parsley or basil on top of your salad before dressing it.

Nutritional Information

Per serving
Total Fat 4g
Net Carbohydrate 1g
Protein 0g

KALE CHIPS (V)

Makes 6 servings (10 chips per serving)

Ingredients

½ pound curly kale leaves
2 tablespoons avocado oil
Sea salt, to taste
Add other spices such as cayenne or cinnamon to spice it up if desired

Instructions

Preheat the oven to 425°F.

Remove the tough stems from the kale. Wash and dry the leaves, then tear into bite-size pieces into a large bowl.

Drizzle the avocado oil over the kale and massage it into the leaves.

Spread the kale leaves evenly on a lined baking sheet and put in the oven. At the 5-minute mark, use a spatula to separate any kale leaves that are sticking together.

Continue baking the kale for about 12 minutes, until the leaves are crisp.

Remove from the oven and sprinkle with salt.

Nutritional Information

Per serving
Total Fat 12g
Net Carbohydrate 2g
Protein 1g

HORMONE FEASTING RECIPES

FLAXSEED-CRUSTED SALMON WITH A ROASTED SQUASH AND BROCCOLI SALAD

Makes 4 servings (2 ounces salmon with ½ cup salad per serving)

Ingredients

Salad

1 small butternut squash, seeds removed, peeled and cubed
4 cups broccoli florets
⅓ cup olive oil, divided
Sea salt
Freshly ground pepper
2 large lemons, juiced and zested
2 tablespoons champagne or white wine vinegar
2 teaspoons Dijon mustard
1 bunch Tuscan kale, washed, stems removed, and chopped
One 14.5-ounce can cannellini or navy beans, drained and rinsed
2 medium Gala apples, cored and sliced thin
1 small shallot, halved and sliced thin
¼ cup roasted pumpkin seeds

Salmon

8-ounce skin-on wild-caught salmon fillet, patted dry
1 teaspoon olive oil
1 teaspoon Dijon mustard
1 garlic clove, grated
2 teaspoons ground flaxseed
2 thyme sprigs, leaves removed and minced

½ teaspoon sea salt
¼ teaspoon freshly ground black pepper

Instructions

Preheat the oven to 400°F.

Line a large rimmed baking sheet with parchment paper, then spread out the squash and broccoli on top. Drizzle 2 to 3 tablespoons of olive oil over the vegetables. Season with salt and pepper and place in the oven.

Roast for 20 to 25 minutes, or until the vegetables are fork tender. Remove from the oven and set aside to cool.

Line a small rimmed baking sheet with parchment paper and place the salmon on top, skin-side down.

Combine the teaspoon of olive oil, mustard, and garlic in a small bowl. Whisk together, then brush evenly over the top and sides of the salmon fillet.

Combine the flaxseed, thyme, salt, and pepper in a separate small bowl. Gently press the mixture into the mustard-glazed flesh of the fish.

Transfer the fish to the oven and bake for about 10 minutes, or until the fish is cooked through and flakes easily with a fork.

While the salmon cooks, finish assembling the salad.

Combine the lemon juice and zest, vinegar, mustard, and remaining olive oil in a small bowl. Whisk together and add salt and pepper to taste.

Combine the kale, beans, apple, shallot, and pumpkin seeds in a large bowl. Add the slightly cooled roasted vegetables. Drizzle the lemony vinaigrette over the top and toss to combine.

Serve the salmon with a large helping of salad.

Nutritional Information

Per serving
Total Fat 27g
Net Carbohydrate 34g
Protein 54g

PUMPKIN CHICKPEA CURRY STEW (V)

Makes 4 servings (1 cup per serving)

Ingredients

2 tablespoons olive oil
1 large onion, diced
8 garlic cloves, minced
1 medium Fresno or jalapeño pepper, seeded and finely chopped
2 tablespoons freshly grated ginger
One 14.5-ounce can pumpkin puree
2 teaspoons ground turmeric
1½ teaspoons sea salt
1 teaspoon cumin
1 teaspoon coriander
1 teaspoon freshly ground black pepper
One 28-ounce can crushed tomatoes
2 to 3 cups vegetable broth
10 ounces fingerling potatoes, quartered
One 14.5-ounce can chickpeas, drained and rinsed
2 cups frozen peas
One 14.5-ounce can full-fat coconut milk

4 cups spinach
1½ cups quinoa, prepared according to the package directions
¼ cup plain coconut milk yogurt
1 lime, cut into wedges

Instructions

Heat the olive oil in a large pot over medium heat. Add the onion and cook for 2 to 3 minutes, or until the onion begins to become translucent. Add in the garlic, pepper, and ginger and stir to combine. Cook for another 2 minutes, stirring gently.

Then stir in the pumpkin puree, turmeric, salt, cumin, coriander, and pepper. Cook for 3 to 5 minutes, or until the mixture becomes fragrant. Add in the tomatoes and 2 cups of broth. Stir everything together, getting all the bits off the bottom of the pot, then add in the potatoes and chickpeas. Stir again, and if the potatoes and beans aren't fully submerged in liquid, slowly add more broth until they're covered.

Bring to a gentle boil, then reduce the heat to low. Cover the pot and simmer for 25 to 30 minutes, or until the potatoes are fork tender.

Once the potatoes are tender, remove the lid and stir in the peas, coconut milk, and spinach. Stir gently over the heat until the spinach wilts. Taste the stew, and add more salt and pepper as needed.

Serve the stew over a scoop of cooked quinoa. Garnish with a dollop of yogurt and a wedge of lime for squeezing on the side.

Nutritional Information

Per serving
Total Fat 16g

Net Carbohydrate 44g
Protein 23g

SESAME GINGER–ROASTED CHICKEN AND SWEET POTATO WITH A FENNEL AND PICKLED BEET SALAD

Makes 4 servings (½ cup chicken on 1½ cups salad per serving)

Ingredients

Chicken and sweet potato

1 tablespoon toasted sesame oil
2 tablespoons avocado oil
¼ cup coconut aminos
2 tablespoons freshly grated ginger
1 teaspoon fish sauce (optional)
4 garlic cloves, minced
1½ teaspoons sea salt
1 teaspoon freshly ground black pepper
One 8-ounce chicken breast, cubed
1 large sweet potato (or 2 medium), peeled and cubed
1 large onion, cut into 1½-inch-thick wedges
1 tablespoon sesame seeds

Salad

¼ cup olive oil
3 tablespoons apple cider vinegar
1 small shallot, minced
Sea salt
Freshly ground black pepper
3 cups arugula
2 cups baby kale

3 small fennel bulbs, trimmed and sliced thin
2 cups pickled beet slices, cut into bite-size pieces
2 cups broccoli slaw mix
2 small Granny Smith apples, cored and sliced thin
2 tablespoons slivered almonds

Instructions

Preheat the oven to 400°F.

Line a rimmed baking sheet with parchment paper.

In a large bowl, combine the first 8 ingredients for the chicken and whisk together well.

Add the cubed chicken, sweet potato, and onion to the bowl with the sesame-ginger mixture and toss to coat evenly.

Scatter the chicken and vegetables evenly on the sheet pan. Reserve any leftover marinade in the bowl. Place the pan in the oven and roast for 15 minutes. Remove the pan from the oven briefly, brushing the chicken and vegetables with the leftover marinade and sprinkling evenly with sesame seeds. Return the pan to the oven and cook for another 20 to 25 minutes, or until the potatoes are fork tender.

While you wait for the chicken and vegetables to finish cooking, prepare the salad.

Whisk together the olive oil, vinegar, and shallot in a small bowl. Season with salt and pepper to taste.

Combine the remaining ingredients in a large serving bowl. When you're ready to serve, toss the salad with the vinaigrette. Serve the salad alongside the roasted chicken and sweet potatoes.

Nutritional Information

Per serving
Total Fat 22g
Net Carbohydrate 56g
Protein 20g

CHIPOTLE BLACK BEAN–STUFFED SWEET POTATOES WITH CILANTRO-LIME CABBAGE SLAW (V)

Makes 4 servings (1 sweet potato over ¾ cup slaw per serving)

Ingredients

Sweet potatoes

4 large sweet potatoes, washed and holes poked with fork or knife
2 tablespoons olive oil
1 red onion, diced
4 ounces tempeh, crumbled
6 garlic cloves, minced
1 chipotle pepper in adobo sauce, finely chopped
One 14.5-ounce can diced tomatoes
One 14.5-ounce can black beans, drained and rinsed
1 cup quinoa, rinsed
2 teaspoons sea salt
1 teaspoon freshly ground black pepper
1 teaspoon cumin
1 teaspoon chili powder
½ teaspoon paprika
¼ teaspoon cayenne pepper

Slaw

2 large limes, juiced
4 tablespoons plain coconut milk yogurt
1 tablespoon avocado oil
2 cups shredded cabbage (green or red)
½ white onion, sliced thin
1 small bunch cilantro, trimmed and chopped
1 avocado, pitted and cubed
Sea salt
Freshly ground black pepper
2 tablespoons ground flaxseeds
2 tablespoons roasted pumpkin seeds

Instructions

Preheat the oven to 425°F.

Line a baking sheet with parchment paper or foil and place the prepared sweet potatoes on top. Bake for about 50 minutes, or until the potatoes are fork tender at the thickest part.

After the sweet potatoes go in the oven, prepare the slaw.

Combine the lime juice, yogurt, and oil in a small bowl. Whisk until combined and set aside.

Combine the cabbage, onion, cilantro, and avocado in a medium or large bowl. Drizzle the lime-coconut mixture over the top and toss to combine. Add salt and pepper to taste, and toss again. Cover the bowl with plastic wrap and place in the refrigerator so the flavors can meld while you finish cooking.

Heat 2 tablespoons of olive oil in a large skillet over medium-high heat. Add in the onion and cook until it starts to become translucent, about 2 to 3 minutes.

Add in the crumbled tempeh and cook until it begins to turn golden. Once the tempeh starts to brown, stir in the minced garlic and cook for another minute, then add in the remaining ingredients (chipotle pepper through cayenne pepper).

Add in 1½ cups of water to give the quinoa enough liquid to cook. Once the mixture begins to boil gently, turn the heat down to medium-low, stirring every so often. Cover and cook for 15 to 20 minutes, or until the sweet potatoes are ready to come out of the oven and the quinoa is beginning to open and curl. If the quinoa-bean mixture begins to boil before the potatoes are done, reduce the heat to its lowest setting to keep the simmer gentle. Taste and adjust the salt and pepper as needed.

Once the sweet potatoes are ready, cut them through the center to release steam, being careful not to cut through the skin on the bottom. Gently pinch the sides to fluff the centers.

Retrieve the slaw from the refrigerator and toss in the flaxseeds and pumpkin seeds.

Serve the potatoes with a generous scoop of both the quinoa-bean mixture and the cilantro cabbage slaw on top.

Nutritional Information

Per serving
Total Fat 18g
Net Carbohydrate 43g
Protein 24g

SHRIMP SCAMPI AND A WARM BACON BALSAMIC SQUASH AND DANDELION SALAD

Makes 4 servings (½ cup scampi with ½ cup each of spaghetti and acorn squash per serving)

Ingredients

Squash

1 large spaghetti squash, halved lengthwise and seeds removed
Olive or avocado oil
1 large acorn squash, halved lengthwise and seeds removed
Sea salt
Freshly ground black pepper

Shrimp

2 tablespoons ghee
8 ounces wild-caught peeled and deveined shrimp
6 minced garlic cloves
1 teaspoon sea salt
1 teaspoon freshly ground black pepper
½ teaspoon red pepper flakes
2 lemons, juiced and zested
1 cup chicken broth
6 cups spinach
1 small bunch parsley, trimmed and chopped

Salad

¼ cup extra-virgin olive oil
3 tablespoons balsamic vinegar
1 tablespoon pure maple syrup
Sea salt
Freshly ground black pepper
2 thick-cut bacon slices, chopped
1 medium shallot, finely diced

4 cups dandelion greens or other bitter green (arugula, kale, radicchio)

1 cup bulgur or quinoa, cooked according to the package directions

¼ cup pomegranate seeds

2 tablespoons roasted sunflower or pumpkin seeds

Instructions

Preheat the oven to 400°F.

Line a large baking sheet with parchment paper.

Lightly grease the flesh of the spaghetti squash with oil, season lightly with salt and pepper, then place on the baking sheet, flesh-side down. Use a fork or a knife to poke a few holes in the top of each half. Place in the oven for 10 minutes.

While the spaghetti squash starts to cook, finish prepping the acorn squash. If you don't like the texture of the skin, peel it now; otherwise just leave it be. Cut each half into ½-inch slices and, as you did with the spaghetti squash, lightly grease all sides of each slice with oil and season lightly with salt and pepper.

After the spaghetti squash gets its 10-minute head start, pull it out of the oven and add the acorn squash to the baking sheet. Return the sheet with both squashes to the oven.

After another 10 to 15 minutes, flip the slices of acorn squash with a spatula, then continue cooking for another 10 to 15 minutes, until both squashes are tender. Once done, remove from the oven, flip the spaghetti squash right side-up so it can release more steam, and set aside.

Begin cooking the shrimp (either while you wait for squash to finish or after it's resting; either works).

Heat the ghee in a large skillet over medium-high heat. Once the ghee is melted, add the shrimp and garlic and season with the salt, pepper, and red pepper flakes. Cook, stirring occasionally, until the shrimp becomes pink and opaque.

Add the lemon juice and zest along with the broth. As soon as the liquids begin to boil, reduce the heat to low. Simmer until the liquids have reduced by half, then stir in the spinach.

After the spinach shrinks and wilts, turn off the heat and gently scoop the cooked flesh from the spaghetti squash into the mixture. The squash's flesh should come apart like pseudo-noodles. Toss the mixture together. Taste and adjust the salt as needed.

Now finish the salad.

Whisk together the oil, vinegar, and maple syrup in a small bowl. Season with salt and pepper to taste and set aside.

Heat a large skillet over medium-high heat. Add the chopped bacon to the pan, stirring occasionally to help each piece cook equally. Once most of the fat is rendered and the bacon is beginning to crisp at the edges, add in the shallot. Cook for another 1 to 2 minutes, or until the shallot becomes translucent.

Turn off the heat and toss in the dandelion greens. Once the greens are just barely wilted, transfer the contents of the skillet to a large bowl. Add in the prepared bulgur, roasted acorn squash, pomegranate seeds, and sunflower seeds. Toss together and then dress with the balsamic vinaigrette.

Serve the scampi with chopped parsley on top and a generous serving of the salad on the side.

Nutritional Information

Per serving
Total Fat 25g
Net Carbohydrate 33g
Protein 47g

GHEE-BASTED PORK CHOPS, SAUTÉED FENNEL, AND LEEKS WITH KALE AND ROASTED POTATOES

Makes 4 servings (1 pork chop and ½ cup vegetables per serving)

Ingredients

Potatoes

1 pound fingerling (or baby) potatoes, washed and halved
2 medium turnips, washed and cubed (about the same size as the halved potatoes)
3 tablespoons ghee, melted
2 garlic cloves, grated
2 rosemary sprigs, leaves removed and minced
1½ teaspoons sea salt
1 teaspoon freshly ground black pepper

Fennel, leeks, and kale

3 tablespoons avocado oil
2 leeks, washed, roots and dark green tops trimmed, white and pale green parts sliced
1 lemon, sliced thin with seeds removed
3 large fennel bulbs, trimmed and sliced thin
1 teaspoon sea salt

1 teaspoon freshly ground black pepper
½ to 1 teaspoon red pepper flakes (½ teaspoon for milder spice, 1 teaspoon if you like more heat)
4 cups kale
1 14.5-ounce can cannellini or navy beans, drained and rinsed

Pork chop

4 thick-cut bone-in pork chops (8 to 10 ounces), patted dry
Sea salt
Freshly ground black pepper
2 fresh thyme sprigs, leaves removed and minced
1 tablespoon ghee, divided
¾ cup chicken broth

Instructions

Preheat the oven to 400°F.

Line a rimmed baking sheet with parchment paper.

Toss together the potatoes and turnips in a large bowl with the ghee, garlic, rosemary, salt, and pepper. Once everything is evenly saturated and seasoned, scatter the potato and turnip mixture evenly onto the prepared baking sheet. Place in the oven and cook for 25 to 30 minutes, or until the vegetables are fork tender.

While the potatoes are roasting, prepare the remaining veggies.

Heat the avocado oil in a large skillet over medium-high heat. Add the leeks and cook for 3 to 4 minutes, or until they start to become tender. Add in the lemon slices and continue cooking for another couple of minutes. Once the leeks are translucent and the lemons are starting to brown at the edges, add in the fennel and season with salt, pepper, and red pepper flakes.

Cook until the fennel starts to shrink and become tender, then add in the kale and beans. Continue cooking for another 3 to 4 minutes, or until the kale wilts and the beans are heated through. Taste, add more salt, if needed, and remove from the heat.

Heat a second skillet over medium-high heat. While the skillet warms, season the pork chops with salt, pepper, and the minced thyme.

Once the skillet is hot, add half of the ghee. After it melts, add in the pork chops. Sear for 5 minutes without touching the pork, then flip them over and sear for another 5 minutes.

After the second side of the pork is done searing, add the remaining ghee to the skillet. Using tongs and a spoon or heat-resistant basting brush, flip the pork chops and glaze with the ghee and cooking juices in the pan. Continue to flip and baste the pork for about 5 minutes, then remove from the skillet and set aside to rest for at least 10 minutes.

Pour the chicken broth into the hot skillet to deglaze it while using a whisk to pull up all the fond (tidbits left from the pork) on the bottom. Once the broth begins to boil, reduce the heat to medium-low and gently boil until the liquid reduces by more than half. Taste the reduction and add more salt if needed.

Slice the pork chops and serve with a big scoop of potatoes, sautéed veggies, and a spoonful of reduction sauce over the top.

Nutritional Information

Per serving
Total Fat 17g
Net Carbohydrate 55g
Protein 26g

CHICKPEA PANCAKES WITH SAUTÉED BEANS AND GREENS WITH A LEMON TAHINI DRESSING (V)

Makes 4 servings (2 pancakes per serving)

Ingredients

Pancakes

4 cups chickpea flour (besan)
⅓ cup nutritional yeast
2 teaspoons sea salt
1 teaspoon freshly ground black pepper
1 teaspoon ground turmeric
1 teaspoon cumin
½ teaspoon coriander
½ teaspoon cayenne pepper
2½ cups water
Avocado oil

Tahini dressing

⅓ cup tahini
1 large lemon, juiced and zested
1 garlic clove, grated
Sea salt
Freshly ground black pepper

Beans and greens

3 tablespoons avocado oil, divided
One 14.5-ounce can chickpeas, drained and rinsed
½ teaspoon sea salt
½ teaspoon freshly ground black pepper
½ teaspoon paprika

½ teaspoon cumin
¼ teaspoon crushed red pepper flakes
3 garlic cloves, grated
6 cups chopped kale

Toppings

1 cup pickled red onion
2 tablespoons toasted sesame seeds
2 tablespoons roasted pumpkin seeds
2 tablespoons whole flaxseeds

Instructions

Combine all the ingredients for the pancakes, except for the oil, in a large bowl. Whisk together until the batter is smooth and no lumps remain, then set aside.

Combine all the ingredients for the tahini dressing in a small bowl. Once combined, slowly drizzle in some water while whisking until the dressing reaches your preferred consistency (you can make it as thick or as thin as you like). Season with salt and pepper to taste and set aside.

Heat 1½ tablespoons of the avocado oil in a large skillet over medium-high heat. Add in the chickpeas, salt, black pepper, paprika, cumin, and red pepper. Cook, stirring occasionally, until the beans begin to turn golden and crispy, then transfer them from the pan and set aside.

Place the remaining 1½ tablespoons of avocado oil in the skillet you used for the beans and return to medium-high heat. Add the garlic and kale and season lightly with salt and pepper. Cook until the kale is wilted, then remove from the heat and set aside.

Heat a small or medium nonstick skillet over medium heat. Add just enough oil to grease the bottom of the pan (less than 1 tablespoon).

Give the resting batter a quick whisk and then scoop out enough batter to nearly coat the bottom of the pan (about ½ cup). Cook the pancake until bubbles begin to appear, 1 to 2 minutes, then gently flip with a spatula and cook for another 2 minutes, or until cooked through and slightly golden. Remove the pancake from the skillet and set aside. Repeat this process until all the batter is used.

Serve the pancakes with the kale and crispy chickpeas on top, drizzle with the tahini dressing, and garnish with pickled onion, sesame seeds, pumpkin seeds, and flaxseeds.

Nutritional Information

Per serving
Total Fat 24.5g
Net Carbohydrate 69g
Protein 33g

WHITE BEAN AND KALE SOUP (V)

Makes 4 servings (1½ cups per serving)

Ingredients

2 tablespoons avocado oil
1 large onion, diced
4 garlic cloves, minced
2 celery stalks, chopped
2 medium carrots, peeled and chopped

2 fresh thyme sprigs, leaves removed and minced
3 fresh oregano sprigs, leaves removed and minced
1½ teaspoons sea salt
1 teaspoon freshly ground black pepper
1 teaspoon crushed red pepper flakes
5 cups vegetable broth
Two 14.5-ounce cans cannellini or navy beans, drained and rinsed
6 cups chopped kale
1 large lemon, cut into wedges

Instructions

Heat the oil in a large pot over medium-high heat. Add the onion and cook for about 2 minutes, or until it starts to become translucent. Add in the next 8 ingredients (garlic through red pepper flakes).

Cook, stirring occasionally, for another 3 minutes, then pour in the broth and beans. Stir together and cook over medium-high heat until the mixture begins to boil.

Reduce the heat to low, taste and add more salt as needed, then cover and simmer for 20 to 25 minutes to allow the flavors to penetrate the beans.

Add the kale to the soup during the last 5 minutes of cooking, stirring well to combine.

Serve the soup with a wedge of lemon to squeeze over the top.

Nutritional Information

Per serving
Total Fat 10g
Net Carbohydrate 48g

Protein 25g

HERBY STEAKS WITH MASHED POTATOES AND ROASTED VEGGIE MEDLEY

Makes 4 servings (2 ounces of steak and ½ cup vegetables per serving)

Ingredients

Steak

10-ounce bone-in ribeye steak
Sea salt
2 teaspoons avocado oil
Freshly ground black pepper
1 tablespoon ghee
1 garlic clove, smashed
1 fresh thyme sprig
1 fresh oregano sprig

Roasted veggies

¼ cup avocado oil
4 cups broccoli florets
4 cups cauliflower florets
4 cups brussels sprouts, trimmed and halved
1½ teaspoons sea salt
1 teaspoon garlic powder
1 teaspoon freshly ground black pepper

Mashed potatoes

1 pound Yukon Gold potatoes, peeled and cubed

Sea salt
3 tablespoons ghee
½ teaspoon ground white pepper (optional)
Freshly ground black pepper

Instructions

Preheat the oven to 400°F.

Line a large baking sheet with parchment paper.

Remove the steak from the refrigerator and season all sides with some salt. Set it aside to rest and come to room temperature.

Combine all the ingredients for the roasted vegetables in a large bowl. Toss together until evenly seasoned and saturated with oil. Transfer to the prepared baking sheet and bake in the oven for 25 to 30 minutes, or until the vegetables are fork tender.

Place the potatoes in a large pot and cover with water. Season the water with salt until it tastes like the sea. Bring to a boil over high heat and cook until the potatoes are fork tender, then remove from stovetop and drain.

Return the strained potatoes to the warm pot they cooked in. Add the ghee, the white pepper, if using, and the black pepper to taste. Mash to desired consistency. The potatoes should be thoroughly seasoned from cooking in the seasoned water, but taste them to be sure and add more salt if needed.

Once the potatoes are done and the roasted vegetables are nearly finished, it's time to cook the steak.

Heat the oil in a medium cast-iron skillet over high heat and finish seasoning the resting steak with some pepper.

Once the skillet is hot and the oil is shimmering, add the steak. Sear the meat without moving it until a nice crust begins to form on the bottom, about 4 to 5 minutes. Turn the steak over and add the ghee, garlic, and herbs.

Using a spoon or heat-resistant basting brush, continuously baste the steak with the garlic-herb ghee while it finishes cooking, another 4 to 5 minutes for medium-rare, or until it reaches your preferred doneness.

Once the steak is done, remove from over the heat and allow it to rest for 10 minutes, then slice and serve with any juices left on the cutting board, along with a generous helping of potatoes and roasted vegetables.

Nutritional Information

Per serving
Total Fat 29g
Net Carbohydrate 27g
Protein 48g

SEED-CRUSTED CAULIFLOWER STEAKS WITH ARUGULA CHIMICHURRI–DRESSED BEANS AND SWEET POTATO FRIES (V)

Makes 4 servings (1 slice cauliflower and ½ cup beans and ½ cup fries per serving)

Ingredients

Chimichurri and beans

2 garlic cloves, smashed

1 small shallot, peeled and roughly chopped
½ teaspoon crushed red pepper flakes
3 cups arugula
1 cup parsley
½ cup olive oil
⅓ cup red wine vinegar
Sea salt
Freshly ground black pepper
One 14.5-ounce can chickpeas, drained (*reserve bean liquid in cans) and rinsed

Fries

1 pound sweet potatoes, peeled and cut into relatively uniform ¼-inch-thick matchsticks
2 tablespoons avocado oil
2 teaspoons pure maple syrup
1 teaspoon cornstarch
1 teaspoon sea salt
1 teaspoon paprika
¼ teaspoon cayenne pepper
Freshly ground black pepper

Cauliflower

⅓ cup nutritional yeast
¼ cup hemp seeds
¼ cup pumpkin seeds
¼ cup ground flaxseed
1 tablespoon chia seeds
2 teaspoons sea salt (use only 1 teaspoon if any of the seeds are pre-salted)
1 teaspoon freshly ground black pepper
1 teaspoon garlic powder
1 teaspoon onion powder
*reserved canned chickpea liquid (aquafaba)

1 large head of cauliflower (or 2 medium), leaves removed, stem trimmed, and cut into 4 "steaks" about 1½ inches thick
2 tablespoons avocado oil

Instructions

Preheat the oven to 425°F.

Line 2 rimmed baking sheets with parchment paper.

First, prepare the chimichurri beans.

Combine the first 5 ingredients in a food processor and pulse until the garlic and shallots are minced and the greens are finely chopped. Add in the olive oil and vinegar, pulsing a few more times until the sauce comes together. Season with salt and pepper to taste.

Combine the chickpeas and chimichurri sauce in a large bowl and toss until the beans are fully saturated, then set aside so the flavors can meld while you finish the rest of the meal. The beans can stay at room temperature or go in the refrigerator if you'd prefer them chilled.

Now prepare the fries.

Combine the sweet potatoes with the oil and syrup in a large bowl and toss together until all the potatoes are fully saturated. Combine the cornstarch, salt, paprika, cayenne, and black pepper in a small bowl. Sprinkle the cornstarch mixture on top of the potatoes. Toss again to distribute evenly; rub the cornstarch into the fries if you see any noticeable streaks of white.

Spread the fries in an even layer on 1 of the prepared baking sheets and place in the oven. Bake for 10 to 15 minutes, then use a spatula to flip the fries over and bake for another 10 to 15 minutes, or until the fries begin to get crispy and golden along the edges.

While the fries bake, prepare the cauliflower.

Combine the first 9 ingredients in a clean food processor and pulse until the seeds form a thick, sandy texture. Transfer the mixture to a small baking sheet (or pie plate) and spread out in an even layer.

Place the reserved aquafaba (chickpea liquids) in a large shallow bowl (or pie plate) and create a small assembly line on your counter. First the bowl with aquafaba, then the seed mixture, and then the second parchment-lined baking sheet.

Now to dredge the cauliflower. Gently take a cauliflower steak and lay it in the aquafaba. Turn it over in the liquid, making sure all the sides are evenly saturated. Transfer the steak to the seed mixture, turning and lightly pressing with your hands to get all the sides covered, then place it on the baking sheet. Repeat this process until all steaks are done.

Gently brush oil over the steaks and place them in the oven. Cook for 15 minutes, then use a spatula to flip them over and cook for another 10 to 15 minutes, or until the cauliflower is tender and the crust is becoming golden brown.

If the fries have lost most of their heat, feel free to pop them in the oven to warm up during the last couple of minutes of the cauliflower cooking time.

Serve the cauliflower steaks with a scoop of the chimichurri chickpeas on top and a helping of sweet potato fries.

Nutritional Information

Per serving

Total Fat 40g
Net Carbohydrate 64g
Protein 24g

QUINOA TABOULI

Makes 6 cups (12 servings, ½ cup per serving)

Ingredients

½ cup quinoa
3 tablespoons lemon juice
2 tablespoons apple cider vinegar
1 tablespoon olive oil
½ teaspoon sea salt
½ teaspoon ground pepper
1 teaspoon ground herbes de Provence
1 cup spinach, chopped
1 cup cherry tomatoes, quartered
1 cup crumbled feta cheese
1 cup red bell pepper, diced

Instructions

Cook the quinoa per the instructions on the package. Fluff and set aside to cool in a large bowl.

While the quinoa is cooking is a perfect time to make the salad dressing with the lemon juice, apple cider vinegar, olive oil, sea salt, pepper, and herbs. Blend evenly and set aside.

Prepare the other ingredients for the salad: Chop the spinach, cut the tomatoes, crumble the feta, and dice the bell peppers.

Once the quinoa has cooled, fluff it again with a fork. Add all the other ingredients, mix to incorporate, and then gently mix in the salad dressing.

Serve at room temperature or refrigerate for a few hours or overnight.

Tips and tricks:

Make sure not to skip the step of rinsing the quinoa before cooking it; this keeps the grains separate and prevents clumps. This recipe tastes even better the next day, so if you're planning a gathering and need to prepare a few things in advance, this salad is a great candidate!

Nutritional Information

Per serving
Total Fat 8g
Net Carbohydrate 5g
Protein 2g

BLACK AND ORANGE RICE

Makes 7 cups (14 servings, ½ cup per serving)

Ingredients

2 cups black rice or wild rice blend
1¾ cups bone broth
4 tablespoons butter
1 cup scallions, thinly sliced (white and light green sections only)
1 cup sliced raw almonds

Zest from 2 medium oranges
6 tablespoons freshly squeezed orange juice
1 teaspoon finely ground pepper
Sea salt to taste

Instructions

Cook the wild rice according to instructions on the package. (This is typically with 2 cups of liquid for every 1 cup of rice, along with the butter, for approximately 45 minutes on simmer after you bring the mixture to a fast boil.) Check on the rice occasionally to make sure the broth is being absorbed evenly.

While the rice is cooking, prepare and measure the other ingredients (zest, juice, sliced scallions, and almonds) and set aside.

When the rice is ready, mix in all the other ingredients and serve.

Nutritional Information

Per serving
Total Fat 4g
Net Carbohydrate 30g
Protein 8g

SWEET POTATO HASH BROWNS

Makes 3 cups (12 servings, ¼ cup per serving)

Ingredients

3 cups shredded sweet potato

1 tablepoon salt (adjust to taste)
1 tablespoon pepper (adjust to taste)
1 teaspoon nutmeg
1 teaspoon allspice
Grass-fed butter

Instructions

Shred the sweet potato with a grater or food processor. (To save time, you can shred the sweet potato in advance; it saves nicely for a few days in the fridge.)

Mix the salt, pepper, nutmeg, and allspice in a medium bowl until evenly combined.

Melt the butter in a frying pan over medium heat. Place several ¼-cup circular mounds of shredded sweet potato in the pan. Cook 4 to 5 minutes on each side, until done. The goal is tender on the inside, slightly crispy on the outside.

Nutritional Information

Per serving
Total Fat 7g
Net Carbohydrate 26g
Protein 3g

ROASTED BUTTERNUT SQUASH SOUP

Makes 6 servings (1 cup per serving)

Ingredients

4 cups butternut squash, cubed and roasted

½ onion, quartered and roasted
½ cup chestnuts, peeled and split in half
2 garlic cloves, smashed
3 tablespoons hazelnut oil
2½ cups bone broth
1 tablespoon raw apple cider vinegar
¼ teaspoon ground ginger
¼ teaspoon ground herbes de Provence
1/8 teaspoon cinnamon
¼ teaspoon salt
1/8 teaspoon pepper
Dash cayenne pepper

Optional garnish

1 tablespoon crème fraîche added to the top of each serving
1 tablespoon fresh thyme, finely minced and sprinkled on each serving

Instructions

Preheat the oven to 350°F.

Seed, peel, and cube the butternut squash and place it in a roasting pan or glass baking dish. Cut the onion half into four wedges and add it to the butternut squash. Stir in the chestnut halves and smashed garlic cloves. Toss the mixture with hazelnut oil and mix in apple cider vinegar, ginger, herbes de Provence, cinnamon, black pepper, and cayenne pepper. Roast for 45 minutes, or until the vegetables are tender and slightly brown.

While the vegetables are roasting, measure out other ingredients.

When the vegetables are ready, let them cool slightly so they're a little easier to handle.

Once the vegetables are cool, transfer them to a food processor or powerful blender. Add the bone broth ½ cup at a time and blend. Continue adding bone broth until the soup is the desired consistency.

Transfer the soup to a large saucepan and bring to a boil. Serve with optional garnishes as desired.

Tips and tricks:

Don't use a roasting pan or baking dish that is too large; keep the vegetables close together so they cook evenly and the smaller pieces don't overcook or burn. Be careful when blending hot foods in a blender or food processor; open lids slowly to avoid an explosion.

Nutritional Information

Per serving
Total Fat 5g
Net Carbohydrate 13g
Protein 2g

CACAO QUINOA CAKE

Makes 8 servings (1 slice per serving, 8 slices per cake)

Ingredients

⅔ cup quinoa
⅓ cup almond milk
1⅓ cups apple sauce

¾ cup coconut oil
2 teaspoons vanilla extract
¼ cup honey
2 eggs
⅓ cup coconut sugar
1 cup raw cacao powder
1½ teaspoons baking powder
½ teaspoon baking soda
½ teaspoon sea salt

Instructions

Cook the quinoa per the package instructions. (Typically, the instructions are to rinse the quinoa grains, boil the grains with 1⅓ cups water, reduce the heat, simmer for 10 minutes, let stand for 10 minutes, and let cool for 15 minutes.)

While the quinoa is cooking, measure all other ingredients and prepare an 8-inch square glass baking pan with coconut oil and oiled parchment paper at the bottom. Set aside.

Once the quinoa is cool enough to handle, preheat the oven to 350°F.

In a food processor, or powerful blender, pulse to blend in 3 stages: First, combine the almond milk, apple sauce, coconut oil, vanilla extract, and honey. Then add the cooked quinoa, eggs, and coconut sugar. Finally, pulse in the cacao powder, baking powder, baking soda, and salt.

Transfer to the baking dish and bake for 1 hour and 25 minutes, or until a toothpick inserted in the center of the cake comes out clean.

Tips and tricks:

This is the moistest gluten-free cake you will ever eat! The final product makes you think there's pudding in the cake. Don't pulse the batter too much; the quinoa in the final baked cake adds to its unique, slightly crunchy texture and helps the cake remain moist.

Nutritional Information

Per serving
Total Fat 1g
Net Carbohydrate 25g
Protein 3g

BREAK YOUR FAST RECIPES

AVOCADO BLUEBERRY SMOOTHIE (V)

Makes 4 servings (12 ounces per serving)

Ingredients

4 cups unsweetened almond milk
2 avocados, pitted and scooped out of skin
4 cups baby spinach
2 cups frozen blueberries
1 cup frozen banana
¼ cup flaxseed

Instructions

Combine all the ingredients in a large blender. Blend until totally smooth and then serve.

Tips and tricks:

If your blender is too small to accommodate all 4 servings, simply make the smoothies in 2 batches.

Nutritional Information

Per serving
Total Fat 32g
Net Carbohydrate 20g
Protein 9g

CHOCOLATEY CHIA FAT BOMBS (V)

Makes 4 servings (2 fat bombs per serving)

Ingredients

⅔ cup almonds
¼ cup almond butter
1 tablespoon coconut oil
1 pitted date
1 teaspoon pure vanilla extract
¼ cup unsweetened shredded coconut
2 tablespoons pumpkin seeds
2 tablespoons chia seeds
1 tablespoon cocoa powder
2 teaspoons cacao nibs
½ teaspoon sea salt

Instructions

Combine all the ingredients in a food processor. Pulse until all the nuts and seeds have mostly broken down and the ingredients begin to come together. Then leave the processor on until the mixture becomes almost smooth, releasing the natural oils and sticking together easily.

Form 8 balls with the fat bomb mixture. Transfer the fat bombs to the refrigerator to firm up for at least 30 minutes before eating.

Store in an airtight container or ziplock bag in the refrigerator (or freezer for more long-term preservation).

Nutritional Information

Per serving
Total Fat 29g
Net Carbohydrate 7g

Protein 8.1g

AVOCADO AND SMOKED SALMON WITH PPP "EVERYTHING BAGEL" SEASONING

Makes 4 servings (½ an avocado and 3 ounces of salmon per serving)

Ingredients

2 large avocados, pitted and scooped out of skin
12 ounces wild-caught smoked salmon
1 small lemon, cut into 4 wedges
4 tablespoons PPP "Everything Bagel" Seasoning (recipe below)

Instructions

Divide the avocado and salmon among 4 plates (½ an avocado and 3 ounces of salmon per plate). Squeeze a wedge of lemon over each serving of avocado and then sprinkle a tablespoon of the seasoning blend over both the avocado and the salmon and serve.

PPP "Everything Bagel" Seasoning

Makes approximately ½ cup

Ingredients

2 tablespoons toasted sesame seeds
1 tablespoon dried minced garlic
1 tablespoon dried minced onion
1 tablespoon flaxseeds

1 tablespoon hemp seeds
2 teaspoons chia seeds
2 teaspoons flaky sea salt (1 teaspoon if using regular fine-ground sea salt)

Instructions

Combine all the ingredients and keep stored in a small airtight container in your pantry.

Give the blend a quick shake or stir before using to help evenly distribute all the delicious components.

Nutritional Information

Per serving
Total Fat 0g
Total Carbohydrate 1g
Protein 0g

FRIED EGGS WITH KIMCHI

Makes 4 servings (2 eggs per serving)

Ingredients

3 tablespoons avocado oil
8 eggs
Sea salt
2 cups kimchi, chopped
Sriracha (optional)

Instructions

Heat the oil in a large nonstick skillet over medium heat. Once the oil starts to shimmer, crack each egg into the pan. Season the eggs lightly with salt.

When you see the egg whites beginning to set, evenly add the kimchi to the pan, trying to avoid scooping it over the yolks so they don't break.

Cook until the egg whites are fully set around the kimchi and the yolks are cooked to your preferred doneness, about 3 to 4 minutes for a runny yolk. Garnish with sriracha if you like.

Nutritional Information

Per serving
Total Fat 10g
Net Carbohydrate 3g
Protein 11g

MIXED-NUT COCONUT FAT BOMBS (V)

Makes 4 servings (2 fat bombs per serving)

Ingredients

⅓ cup pecans
⅓ cup hazelnuts
¼ cup almond butter
1 tablespoon coconut oil
1 pitted date
1 teaspoon pure vanilla extract
1 tablespoon flaxseeds
1 tablespoon hemp seeds
1 tablespoon chia seeds

½ teaspoon cinnamon
½ teaspoon cardamom
½ teaspoon salt
½ cup unsweetened shredded coconut

Instructions

Combine all the ingredients, except for the shredded coconut, in a food processor. Pulse until all the nuts and seeds have mostly broken down and the ingredients begin to come together. Then leave the processor on until the mixture becomes almost smooth, releasing the natural oils and sticking together easily.

Scatter the shredded coconut in an even layer on a large plate. Form 8 balls with the fat bomb mixture. Roll each ball in the shredded coconut and then transfer them to the refrigerator to firm up for at least 30 minutes before eating.

Store in an airtight container or ziplock bag in the refrigerator (or freezer for more long-term preservation).

Nutritional Information

Per serving
Total Fat 32g
Net Carohydrate 6g
Protein 6g

BURGER PATTY WITH GUACAMOLE

Makes 4 servings (1 burger per serving)

Ingredients

Burgers

1 pound ground beef
2 tablespoons avocado oil, divided
1 tablespoon coconut aminos
1 egg, lightly beaten
¼ cup almond meal
1 small onion, finely chopped
3 garlic cloves, grated
1 teaspoon sea salt
1 teaspoon freshly ground black pepper

Guacamole

½ small red onion, roughly chopped
1 small jalapeño, seeded and roughly chopped
1 medium heirloom or vine-ripened tomato, roughly chopped
½ cup cilantro *corriander*
2 avocados, pitted and scooped out of skins
1 lime, cut into wedges
Sea salt

Instructions

Combine all the ingredients for the burgers in a large bowl (just reserve 1 of the tablespoons of oil).

Using clean hands, combine all the ingredients for the burgers thoroughly, then set aside for the flavors to meld while you prepare the guacamole.

Place the onion, jalapeño, tomato, and cilantro in a food processor and pulse until the mixture is roughly diced. Transfer the mixture to a large bowl with the avocado.

Mash the avocado and onion mixture using a fork until it reaches your preferred consistency—chunky, smooth, or somewhere in between.

Stir in the juice from a couple of lime wedges, season with salt to taste, then set aside and cook the burgers.

Heat the reserved tablespoon of oil in a large cast-iron skillet over medium-high heat. While the cast iron heats, form 4 patties. Once the oil begins to shimmer, place the burgers in the skillet. Cook for 4 to 5 minutes per side, or until cooked to your preferred doneness.

Serve the burgers with a generous scoop of guacamole on top and a wedge of lime.

Nutritional Information

Per serving
Total Fat 26g
Net Carbohydrate 7g
Protein 39g

VANILLA BEAN CHIA PUDDING WITH BERRIES AND CHOCOLATE (V)

Makes 4 servings (½ cup per serving)

Ingredients

2 cups full-fat coconut milk
2 teaspoons vanilla bean paste or extract
¼ cup chia seeds
Pinch of salt

Toppings

2 cups fresh berries of your choice
4 ounces vegan 70 percent dark chocolate

Instructions

Combine all the ingredients for the chia pudding in a medium mixing bowl. Transfer the mixture to a container with a fitted lid and place in the refrigerator. For the first 30 minutes, stir the pudding every 10 minutes so the seeds distribute evenly while it sets up.

Allow the pudding to gel in the refrigerator for at least 2 hours or overnight.

Serve the pudding topped with the berries of your choice. For the finishing touch, grate the dark chocolate over each serving.

Nutritional Information

Per serving
Total Fat 12g
Net Carbohydrate 14g
Protein 4g

TUNA SALAD–STUFFED AVOCADO

Makes 4 servings (1 avocado half per serving)

Ingredients

Two 4-ounce cans tuna packed in oil
¼ cup keto-approved mayonnaise

1 lemon, juiced and zested
1 medium shallot, finely chopped
2 tablespoons freshly chopped dill
Sea salt
Freshly ground black pepper
2 large avocados, pitted and halved with skin left on
2 cups fermented vegetables of your choosing, such as dill pickles, kimchi, or curtido, etc.

Instructions

Combine the first 5 ingredients in a medium mixing bowl. Use a fork to flake the tuna and fully incorporate it with the other ingredients. Season with salt and pepper to taste.

Divide the tuna salad evenly among the 4 open-face avocado halves. Serve each stuffed avocado with ½ cup of fermented veggies on the side.

Nutritional Information

Per serving
Total Fat 23g
Net Carbohydrate 3g
Protein 6g

STRAWBERRY MINT KEFIR SMOOTHIE (V)

Makes 4 servings (12 ounces per serving)

Ingredients

4 cups raw kefir
2 cups frozen strawberries

1 cup frozen banana
8 to 10 fresh mint leaves
2 tablespoons hemp seeds
2 tablespoons chia seeds

Instructions

Combine all the ingredients in a large blender. Blend until totally smooth and serve.

If your blender is too small to accommodate all 4 servings, simply make the smoothies in 2 batches.

Nutritional Information

Per serving
Total Fat 6g
Net Carbohydrate 24g
Protein 12g

GARLICKY CIDER SPINACH WITH JAMMY EGGS

Makes 4 servings (1 cup per serving)

Ingredients

8 eggs
2 tablespoons ghee
6 garlic cloves, minced
8 cups spinach
2 tablespoons apple cider vinegar
Sea salt
Freshly ground black pepper

Instructions

Bring a large pot of water to a rolling boil over high heat, then reduce the heat to medium so the water simmers down to a gentle boil.

Gently lower the eggs into the water using a slotted spoon and cook for 7 to 7½ minutes. While the eggs are in the pot, fill a large bowl with ice and cold water.

Immediately transfer the cooked eggs to the ice bath to prevent further cooking while you prepare the spinach.

Heat the ghee in a large skillet over medium-high heat. Once the oil begins to shimmer, add the garlic and cook for 30 seconds, then add the spinach and vinegar. Cook and stir until the spinach is fully wilted and the moisture released from the leaves reduces by half. Turn off the heat and season the spinach with salt and pepper to taste.

Peel the eggs, cut them in half, and season them lightly with a pinch of salt.

Divide the spinach among 4 bowls and top each with 2 eggs (4 halves).

Nutritional Information

Per serving
Total Fat 15g
Net Carbohydrate 3g
Protein 13g

SPICED COCONUT CURRY HUMMUS (V)

Makes 3½ cups (28 servings, 2 tablespoons per serving)

Ingredients

6 cups chickpeas, drained
2 garlic cloves
2 tablespoons coconut manna
2 tablespoons tahini
¼ cup lime juice
4 tablespoons water
1 teaspoon garlic powder
8 teaspoons yellow curry powder
½ teaspoon ground turmeric
4 teaspoons honey
⅓ cup olive oil
Sea salt and pepper to taste
2 tablespoons shredded coconut, unsweetened
½ cup jalapeño, finely diced

Instructions

Combine everything except the shredded coconut and jalapeño in a powerful blender. If the mixture is too thick, add more water and/or olive oil.
Once the desired consistency is achieved, spoon in the shredded coconut and diced jalapeño.

Tips and tricks:

This hummus is sweet and spicy, with a big kick. It serves well as a dip with seeded crackers and raw vegetables such as jicama, bell pepper, and carrots.

Nutritional Information

Per serving

Total Fat 3g
Net Carbohydrate 3g
Protein 1g

COCONUT CACAO CHIA PUDDING (V)

Makes approximately 4½ cups (13 servings, ⅓ cup per serving)

Ingredients

3 cups coconut milk
⅔ cup chia seeds
½ cup raw cacao powder
1 teaspoon vanilla extract
½ teaspoon sea salt
1 teaspoon ground cinnamon (optional)
⅓ cup maple syrup (optional)

Instructions

Combine all the ingredients, including the cinnamon and maple syrup, if using, in a large mixing bowl and blend vigorously.

Chill in the fridge between 3 hours and overnight. The goal is for the mixture to have a pudding-like consistency and to be chilled through.

Leftovers keep covered in the fridge for 2 to 3 days, though this pudding is best when it's fresh.

Serve chilled.

Serving suggestion:

Top with coconut yogurt, raw almonds, raspberries, blueberries, shaved coconut flakes, and finely sliced mint leaves.

Nutritional Information

Per serving
Total Fat 9g
Net Carbohydrate 6g
Protein 3g

PUMPKIN SPICE SPREAD (V)

Makes 2½ cups (20 servings, 2 tablespoons per serving)

Ingredients

1 cup raw pumpkin seeds
1 cup almond flour
¾ cup pumpkin puree
½ cup pumpkin oil (use less for a thicker consistency)
1 tablespoon lemon juice
2 teaspoons cinnamon
1 teaspoon cardamom
2 tablespoons plus 1 teaspoon honey
½ teaspoon cloves
Freshly ground nutmeg
1 cup grated green apple

Instructions

Place the pumpkin seeds in a powerful blender and pulse until they are finely ground.

Add in the remaining ingredients and blend to your desired consistency.

Transfer the spread to a glass storage container; it will keep in the fridge for 5 to 7 days.

Tips and tricks:

If the spread is too thick, add a small amount of almond milk. If the spread is too thin, add more almond flour.

Nutritional Information

Per serving
Total Fat 25g
Net Carbohydrate 3g
Protein 2g

BASIC BEEF BONE BROTH

Makes 6 to 8 cups (approximately 1 cup per serving)

Ingredients

2 pounds grass-fed beef bones
2 tubers of organic turmeric, cut into large pieces
3 organic garlic cloves, peeled
1 medium onion, cut into large cubes
2 tablespoons apple cider vinegar

Instructions

Wash the bones and place them in the bottom of a slow cooker.

Add the turmeric pieces, whole garlic cloves, and onions to the bones.

Add enough water to fill to the top of the slow cooker, then add in the apple cider vinegar.

Set on medium heat for the first hour. Periodically watch for any foam that might appear at the beginning of cooking. Scrape this foam off as you see it form.

After 1 hour, turn down the heat to low and let the broth cook for 48 hours before you drink it.

Tips and tricks:

The quality of the bones is one of the most important aspects of this wonderful broth. If you use chicken, making this broth takes bones from 2 to 3 chickens. Chicken feet are also great to use, as they create a more healing, gelatinous soup.

Nutritional Information

Per serving
Total Fat 14g
Net Carbohydrate 0g
Protein 18g

Afterword

I am going to let you in on a little secret. I didn't set out to be a fasting expert. In fact, in my early years in undergraduate school I thought I wanted to be a journalist. Then I sat in an anatomy class and my obsession with the human body was birthed. The more I learn, the more in awe I am of just how well designed this beautiful home is that carries us around every day.

Many doctors will tell you that they learn so much from their patients. I definitely fit into that camp. My passion for the past 26 years has been fueled by the people I serve and their desire to use their lifestyle as a healing tool. I remember early on in my career, a woman named Lani came to my office who at 40 years old walked into her ob-gyn's office for a routine mammogram and came out with a diagnosis of metastatic breast cancer. She was given three months to live. With persistence and a whole lot of tenacity, she turned that three-month prognosis into 11 years, largely by changing her lifestyle. I feel so honored to have intimately walked that healing path with her, and to have witnessed firsthand how dramatically influential one's health habits can be in challenging a deadly prognosis. Months before she passed, Lani asked me what I knew about the healing effects of fasting. At that time, I knew nothing about fasting. It was her curiosity to learn this healing tool that sparked my decade-long fascination with the research on fasting. I wish she were alive today for me to show her what I've discovered.

Lani had a heart for serving her community. As she learned how her lifestyle choices contributed to her cancer diagnosis, she turned around and educated everyone in her community. She so desperately wanted others to know what caused a body to fall prey to cancer. In her final months while in hospice care, I asked Lani how I could best carry her message forward. Her response to me was, "Mindy, people will never get healthy until they are willing to do the work." The day she died, my mission to teach the world how to do the work began.

As my conviction for fasting grew, the more vocal I became. Social media became my outlet to amplify my fasting message to the world. The more I educated the masses, the more healing stories poured in. Every week thousands of fasting testimonials have appeared on my social platforms. These stories have touched my soul in the deepest way and continue to prove that fasting is a tool that can be used by anyone, anywhere, for healing. It doesn't matter how much money you have or time available, fasting will work for you.

In March 2020, when the pandemic first hit, much like many of you, I was in shock. Soon my shock moved to awe that the whole world was going to start paying attention to their health now. The world was ready to do the work. As I scoured the newly emerging studies revealing the comorbidities that were causing people to fall prey to this new virus, it became extremely clear that poor metabolic health was at the root of an immune-compromised body. Fasting as a free tool for metabolic health became my creed. If we all rallied around the idea that a healthy, functioning immune system begins with great metabolic health, we could gain some health control in a world that feels like it's spinning out of control. Yet as I write this, we are almost two years into this pandemic with very little front-page news or direction from leaders on the responsibility we play in cleaning up our own metabolic profile. This saddens me deeply as there is so much personal responsibility we can take in this moment.

We have many historical examples of progress that has emerged from troubled times. Out of the 1918 pandemic flu emerged the Roaring '20s. From the sorrow of a two-year deadly pandemic mixed with the end of a war emerged a time of celebration and community. People reevaluated what was important to them. Isolation was transformed into social connection. One of the symbolic themes of this time was "The New Woman"—a less ladylike, more unruly version of a woman that the world had never seen. At this moment in our current history, we are ready for a new woman to reemerge. This time she's going to be "The Empowered Woman," a woman who is filled with faith for her health, not fear. A woman who won't be given a one-size-fits-all approach to her life. A woman who gathers the support of other women around her to build each other up. This is our moment to create a new path. But it's going to require you to put down the feelings of guilt that may flood your mind from failed diets. You can't step into this empowered state with remnants of shame left over from poor lifestyle choices. You can't bring hate for your body on this next leg of your health journey. And it will behoove you to stop comparing yourself to other women as you watch their highlight reels on social media. It's time as women that we lean in to each other, create communities that lift each other up, and see that collaboration, not competition, is where we shine best.

Fasting like a girl will be an integral part of this new emergence for women. As more women use the principles I've laid out in this book, you will see a world in which women unite in health and love for one another. I know fasting can dramatically change the metabolic health of women without them having to spend a dime. I dream of a time when communities of women fast together not only to improve their health but for spiritual and emotional connection with each other. It's our time now. We don't have to play by the old rules. We get to create something new that the world has never seen before. Take pride in this new empowered place from which you will grow. Support other women to do the same. Together we will rise. In love. In compassion for one another. And in health. I love being on this journey with all of you. Massive gratitude to you all.

Appendix A

Glossary of Most-Used Fasting Terms

In this book, there may be lots of terms that are new to you. At first these terms can be confusing, but as you learn to fast like a girl, you will see that fasters worldwide refer to these terms often, so it's good to familiarize yourself with them.

Apoptosis: The death of cells that occurs as a normal and controlled part of an organism's growth or development.

Autophagy: Autophagy is the natural, regulated mechanism of the cell that removes unnecessary or dysfunctional components. It allows the orderly degradation and recycling of cellular components. Triggered by a decline in the influx of nutrients into a cell, this self-repair process often begins when your cells sense a decline in nutrients. This can happen after 17 hours of fasting and will peak at 72 hours of fasting.

Blood sugar: The amount of glucose that is readily circulating in your blood. Healthy blood sugar should be between 70 and 90 mg/dL (milligrams per deciliter) when in a fasted state.

Breaking a fast: A common term used to refer to a food or drink that raises your blood sugar, thus turning off the healing switches and pulling you out of a fast.

Eating window: The time period in your 24-hour day when you are eating. Typically, your eating window is marked by an increase in blood sugar.

Fasting window: The time period in your 24-hour day when you are not eating. Any food or drink that raises your blood sugar will pull you out of your fasted window. Most fasted windows are greater than 13 hours.

Fat-adapted: An energy system that your body taps into in the absence of food, specifically carbohydrates. Ketones are a signal that the body is now operating from a fat-adapted place.

Fat burner: An energy system that burns fuel from your fat.

Insulin resistance: A state in which a person's body has a lowered level response to insulin, impairing the ability for glucose to enter the cells.

Intermittent fasting: Going without food for 13 to 15 hours.

Ketones: The signal that your liver is now burning energy from fat, not sugar. Healthy ketone range typically is .5–6.0 mmol/L (millimoles per liter).

Ketosis: A process that happens when your body doesn't have enough carbohydrates to burn for energy. Instead, it burns fat and makes ketones, which it can use for fuel.

Metabolic flexibility: A term used to indicate your ability to easily switch back and forth from sugar burner to fat burner.

Metabolic switching: The body's ability to switch back and forth between the sugar-burning and fat-burning energy systems.

Mitochondria: Surrounded by a bilipid membrane, this is the part inside your cells that provides you with energy, called ATP, and produces glutathione for detoxification.

mTOR: A cellular signaling pathway that gets triggered when amino acids and insulin levels within the cell increase. Usually this happens from an influx of protein. Once stimulated, the mTOR pathway will promote cellular growth.

OMAD: A common term used among fasters to indicate they are eating only one meal a day.

Protein synthesis: A natural process that your body is dependent upon to perform daily functions, create enzymes, and build structural support. Essential amino acids from your diet are needed in order for this process to occur.

Stored sugar: The amount of glucose that is stored in tissues like the liver, fat, brain, and eyes. There is no real measurement of stored sugar.

Sugar burner: An energy system that burns fuel from the foods you eat.

Water fasting: A fast that involves drinking only water. Most water fasts are three days or longer.

Appendix B

Food Lists

Intentionally eating foods that support your hormonal health can be tricky at first. As a culture, we have been conditioned to choose our foods based on what our taste buds like. To help keep you focused on nourishing your body with the best foods possible, I have broken down the following list into foods that support your hormones, microbiome, and liver, as well as those that help you build muscle.

A few things to keep in mind as you read through this list. First, this is a starting point to help you understand which foods you can lean in to to support different aspects of your health. As you learn more about customizing a fasting lifestyle that's unique to you, you may find new foods that fall into one of these categories that I didn't list. That's okay. The list is meant to get you in the ballpark. Second, you will see that some foods overlap into multiple categories—that just means these are hormonal superpower foods. Cruciferous vegetables like brussels sprouts and broccoli are great for estrogen, progesterone, and gut and liver health. Feel free to eat these vegetables all month long. Third, because pesticides are a known endocrine disruptor that can wreak hormonal havoc on you, try to get these foods organic, non-GMO, and antibiotic-free whenever possible.

Lastly, I want to point out that each list of food plays a part in the two food plans I mapped out for you in the 30-Day Fasting Reset. Along with each list, I note which plan those foods fall into. To remind you of the macros of each of those food plans, I have outlined them below.

Have fun experimenting with all of these delicious foods. Be sure to also try out the recipes included in this book that bring many of these foods to life. Happy hormone fueling!

KETOBIOTIC FOOD PLAN

- 50 grams net carbohydrates
- 75 grams protein
- >60 percent of your food coming from good fat

HORMONE FEASTING FOOD PLAN

- 100–150 grams net carbohydrates
- 50 grams protein
- Healthy fats as desired

ESTROGEN-BUILDING FOODS

These foods work well for ketobiotic days. You will want to put your food focus on these foods during your two power phases (days 1–10 and 16–19 of your cycle).

Seeds and Nuts

- Brazil nuts
- Almonds
- Cashews
- Roasted salted peanuts
- Pine nuts

- Pumpkin seeds
- Sunflower seeds
- Walnuts
- Sesame seeds

Legumes

- Peas
- Chickpeas
- Soybeans
- Lima beans
- Carob
- Kidney beans
- Mung beans
- Pinto beans
- Black-eyed peas
- Lentils

Fruits and Vegetables

- Cabbage
- Spinach
- Sprouts
- Onions
- Garlic
- Zucchini
- Broccoli

- Cauliflower
- Strawberries
- Blueberries
- Cranberries

PROGESTERONE-BUILDING FOODS

These foods are perfect for the hormone feasting food plan. You want to put your food focus on these foods during the manifestation and nurture phases (days 11–15 and 20–30 respectively). If weight loss is your focus, be sure to keep closer to 100 grams of net carbohydrates on these days.

Root Vegetables

- White potatoes
- Red potatoes
- Sweet potatoes
- Yams
- Beets
- Turnips
- Fennel
- Pumpkin
- Butternut squash
- Acorn squash
- Honeynut squash
- Spaghetti squash

Cruciferous Vegetables

- Brussels sprouts
- Cauliflower
- Broccoli

Tropical Fruits

- Bananas
- Mangoes
- Papaya

Citrus Fruits

- Oranges
- Grapefruit
- Lemons
- Limes

Seeds

- Sunflower
- Flax
- Sesame

Legumes

- Chickpeas
- Kidney beans
- Black beans

The three Ps—probiotic, prebiotic, and polyphenol foods—and bitter foods are great throughout your cycle, but they're especially important during your manifestation phase (days 11–15 of your cycle).

PROBIOTIC-RICH FOODS

- Sauerkraut
- Kimchi
- Pickles
- Yogurt
- Kefir

POLYPHENOL FOODS

- Broccoli
- Shallots
- Brussels sprouts
- Parsley
- Artichoke hearts
- Olives
- Red wine
- Dark chocolate

PREBIOTIC FOODS

- Chicory root
- Dandelion root

- Konjac root
- Burdock root
- Onions
- Jerusalem artichokes
- Garlic
- Leeks
- Asparagus
- Red kidney beans
- Chickpeas
- Split peas
- Cashews
- Pistachios
- Hummus

BITTER FOODS THAT SUPPORT LIVER HEALTH

- Arugula
- Coffee
- Dill
- Dandelion greens
- Jerusalem artichokes
- Brussels sprouts
- Eggplant
- Saffron
- Kale
- Sesame seeds

- Turmeric
- Ginger
- Citrus such as lemons, limes, and grapefruit
- Peppermint
- Green tea

GOOD, HEALTHY FATS

Good fats are important throughout your menstrual cycle, so feel free to eat these all month long. You will find good fats especially helpful on ketobiotic days as hunger can creep in because of the lower carbohydrate count. Remember, good fats kill hunger, so seek out these yummy fats when your brain wants more food.

- Olive oil
- Avocado oil
- Coconut oil
- MCT oil
- Sesame oil
- Flaxseed oil
- Black cumin oil
- Coriander oil
- Avocados
- Olives
- Coconut
- Raw nut butters
- Grass-fed dairy

- Grass-fed butter

MUSCLE-BUILDING FOODS

Integrating these proteins into your diet all month long will help you build muscle. Remember that as you age, your amino acid nutrient sensors in your muscles become less efficient. If you want to build more muscle, then make sure you are getting at least 25 grams of protein at one meal to trigger those sensors.

- Quinoa
- Eggs
- Turkey
- Chicken
- Cottage cheese
- Mushrooms
- Fish
- Shellfish
- Red meat such as lamb and beef
- Pork
- Chia seeds
- Tofu

Appendix C

Fasting Protocols to Help Specific Conditions

Over the years, my patients have used many fasting lifestyle variations with great success. Below are my tried-and-true fasting protocols. If you are struggling with any of the health concerns listed, I highly recommend you do the 30-Day Fasting Reset first to get the foundational experience of what it is like to fast like a girl. After that you can move on to the protocols I outline. Regardless of the protocol you choose, it's best to involve your doctor in this fasting journey with you.

INFERTILITY

There are many reasons a woman can be infertile. In fact, in today's world one out of every eight women will become infertile. That statistic alone is daunting and should give you insight into the root cause of infertility. Women are all living in the same modern world, engaging in similar habits (such as eating all day; eating processed, quick, grab-and-go foods that are full of toxins; not paying attention to our sleep or stress; moving less than we were designed to; and ignoring our hormonal lenses). This is leading so many women to one condition: insulin resistance.

In order for your sex hormones to function normally, you need to be sensitive to insulin. As long as you are in a state of insulin resistance, your sex hormones will struggle. I know I keep saying this over and over again, but this is such a key point I want you to get. I watch women spend thousands of dollars on

IVF treatment without taking the first free step—fixing their lifestyle. Nothing will fix insulin resistance like a fasting lifestyle.

This fasting protocol was built out of necessity. Several of my patients were struggling with fertility issues, so I wanted to create a fasting lifestyle that would help balance insulin and amplify sex hormones. I knew that a couple of months of varying their fasts and food would help. This fasting variation worked so well for infertility that it has now become my go-to for women looking for lifestyle solutions to their fertility hurdles.

2-month fasting protocol for infertility

Month 1

Days 1–3: 15 hours intermittent fasting (ketobiotic)
Days 4–10: 17 hours autophagy fasting (ketobiotic)
Days 11–15: 13 hours intermittent fasting (hormone feasting)
Days 16–19: 13 hours intermittent fasting (ketobiotic)
Day 20–bleed (through day 28): no fasting (hormone feasting)

Month 2

Days 1–5: 17 hours autophagy fasting (ketobiotic)
Day 6: 24 hours gut-reset fast (ketobiotic)
Days 7–10: 17 hours autophagy fasting (ketobiotic)
Days 11–15: 13 hours intermittent fasting (hormone feasting)
Day 16–bleed: no fasting (hormone feasting)

AUTOIMMUNE CONDITIONS: RHEUMATOID ARTHRITIS, LUPUS, HASHIMOTO'S, PCOS

When it comes to an autoimmune condition, I want you to think of two aspects of your health: your gut and your toxic load. These two are at the core of why you are not feeling well. The exciting part is that we can help both of these imbalances with a fasting lifestyle. Knowing that toxins and gut imbalances are at the root of all autoimmune conditions, there are two fasts that will help you tremendously: gut reset (24 hours) and autophagy (17 hours). This doesn't mean you do these fasts all month long, but you will definitely want to cycle them into your monthly fasting regime. Here is an example of a monthlong fasting protocol that can help with autoimmune conditions. If the longer fasts feel like a stretch for you, be sure you do the 30-Day Fasting Reset for a couple of months before you go to this advanced autoimmune protocol.

Fasting protocol for autoimmunity

Days 1–5: 17 hours autophagy fasting (ketobiotic)
Days 6–7: 24 hours gut-reset fast (ketobiotic)
Days 8–10: 17 hours autophagy fast (ketobiotic)
Days 11–15: 15 hours intermittent fasting (hormone feasting)
Days 16–17: 24 hours gut-reset fast (ketobiotic)
Days 18–19: 17 hours autophagy fasting (ketobiotic)
Day 20–bleed: 13 hours intermittent fasting (hormone feasting)

THYROID CONDITIONS

When you look at building a fasting lifestyle that will help your thyroid problems, you have to take into consideration all the organs that need to be healthy in order for your thyroid to function properly. When it comes to our endocrine glands, like the thyroid, there is a team of organs that assist in the production, metabolism, and utilization of the hormones needed to allow that gland to do its job. For the thyroid, the brain, liver, and gut need to be working properly.

When I say, "brain," you say, "autophagy." With all thyroid conditions, you want to use the autophagy tool as much as possible. As you know, autophagy fasting is best done in your power phases. When supporting the liver, you want to incorporate hormone feasting foods with plenty of cruciferous and bitter greens.

Fasting protocol for thyroid conditions

Days 1–5: 15 hours intermittent fasting (ketobiotic)
Days 6–8: 17 hours autophagy fasting (ketobiotic)
Days 9–10: 24 hours gut-reset fast (ketobiotic)
Days 11–15: 15 hours intermittent fasting (hormone feasting foods)
Days 16–19: 17 hours autophagy fasting (ketobiotic)
Day 20–bleed: 13 hours intermittent fasting (hormone feasting)

CHRONIC FATIGUE

Like many of the conditions I have mentioned here, there can be multiple causes, but the three most common causes of chronic fatigue are depleted cellular mitochondria, adrenal exhaustion, and Epstein-Barr virus. My chronic fatigue was because of the latter. Knowing the root cause of your chronic fatigue can be extremely helpful, but if you are unsure of its origin, no worries, going through the protocol I give below will help.

Your mitochondria are the part of your cells that give you energy. They become depleted for a variety of reasons, but the main ones are too many toxins, eating the wrong oils, and consuming a highly refined carbohydrate diet. Sound familiar? Yep, that's the standard American diet. If you are chronically fatigued and need to eat all day long, there is a good chance that you have depleted mitochondria, and the good news is that your mitochondria heal with ketones, so the protocol I take you through below will help greatly.

If you know you are adrenal exhausted, I encourage you to look below at the protocol for adrenal fatigue. Lastly, if you have been tested for Epstein-Barr virus and know that you have high amounts, the key fasting principle to know here is that one way to stop viral replication is to have your cells operating from your fat-burning energy pathways the majority of the time. When you're doing the longer fasts, a diet low in carbohydrates will be best. You will see that I have lots of low-carb living in this protocol.

Fasting protocols for chronic fatigue

Days 1–3: 13 hours intermittent fasting (ketobiotic)
Days 4–6: 15 hours intermittent fasting (ketobiotic)
Day 7: 17 hours autophagy fasting (ketobiotic)
Days 8–9: 15 hours intermittent fasting (ketobiotic)
Days 10–15: 13 hours intermittent fasting (hormone feasting foods)
Days 16–19: 15 hours intermittent fasting (ketobiotic)
Day 20–bleed: no fasting (hormone feasting)

TYPE 2 DIABETES

The first thing I want to emphasize if you are a diabetic who is building a fasting lifestyle is to be sure that you include your doctor in this conversation. I have a great YouTube video called "Why Your Doctor Should Be Recommending Intermittent Fasting" that links to one of the largest meta-analyses done on fasting, published in *The New England Journal of Medicine*. We want your doctor on your fasting team so that you can thrive with your health.

As you most likely know, the root cause of type 2 diabetes is insulin resistance, which makes building a fasting lifestyle quite simple. Although metabolic switching is always the goal, you'll want to spend more time as a fat burner. This means that monitoring your blood sugar and insulin levels is key. You will also notice that I did not include a hormone-building day in the fasting protocol. The reason is that you want to keep away from the higher-carbohydrate feast days. As your blood sugar stabilizes, you can switch out the protein-load day for a hormone-building day, but be sure you are getting great blood sugar readings for several months in a row before you do that. Again, involving your doctor in this conversation is critical.

Fasting protocol for type 2 diabetes

Days 1–5: 13 hours intermittent fasting (ketobiotic)
Days 6–10: 15 hours intermittent fasting (ketobiotic)
Days 11–15: 13 hours intermittent fasting (hormone feasting)
Day 16: 17 hours autophagy fasting (ketobiotic)
Days 17–19: 13 hours intermittent fasting (ketobiotic)
Day 20–bleed: no fasting (hormone feasting)

BRAIN HEALTH: MEMORY LOSS, DEPRESSION, ANXIETY

When you get gaps in memory, whether or not you are predisposed to Alzheimer's, lose words, have trouble focusing, or chunks of your memory are starting to slip away, a fasting lifestyle can help. If you haven't heard that Alzheimer's is diabetes of the brain, then I want to bring this to your attention. The reason it's so important is insulin resistance is at the root of so many of the conditions plaguing humans today. This is why, first and foremost, we all have to learn how to manage insulin better, and fasting does that for us.

The other side of the memory issue involves toxins, heavy metals specifically. Heavy metals will block receptor sites on the ends of neurons, slowing the transmission of information across your brain neurons, leaving you with gaps of information. Heavy metals are all over our environment. They are in our soils, air, water, foods, beauty products, cleaning products, and even in the fish we eat. When I look at the epidemic of Alzheimer's cases we have and hear stories of people in their 50s and 60s getting Alzheimer's, I become more and more convinced that a fasting lifestyle would help dramatically.

Knowing that toxins and mismanaged blood sugar and insulin are at the root of so many memory problems, we can now lean in to our fasting principles. Once again, with mismanaged insulin I want to make sure you stay in fat-burning mode as much as possible while using the principles of autophagy to clean up the dysfunctional neurons in your brain. Also keep in mind that ketones are healing to the brain, so you want to make lots of those to accelerate the healing that needs to happen to get your brain back on track.

If you are experiencing mood disorders like depression or anxiety, be assured that as ketones go up, so do neurotransmitters like GABA, serotonin, and dopamine. Often the longer you fast, the more ketones your body will make. You will see I included a long, 48-hour dopamine fast in this protocol. Also keep in mind that minerals are key for mood disorders like depression, so increasing your mineral supplementation is pivotal.

Here's what a good protocol for brain health would look like.

Fasting protocol for memory loss

Days 1–5: 17 hours autophagy fasting
Days 6–7: 48 hours dopamine fasting
Days 8–10: 15 hours intermittent fasting
Days 11–15: 13 hours intermittent fasting

Days 16–19: 17 hours autophagy fasting
Day 20–bleed: 13 hours intermittent fasting

ADRENAL FATIGUE

If you are adrenal fatigued, I want you to remember to slow your way into fasting. I am making some modifications to the timing around the fasts for this protocol, so pay close attention to the hours I put next to each fast. The other key to building a fasting lifestyle for those who are adrenal fatigued is making sure you increase your good fat. You will want to stabilize your blood sugar to make fasting easier. The worst thing someone with adrenal fatigue could do when they fast is eat a high-carbohydrate, low-fat diet; this will make fasting incredibly hard, if not impossible.

The other key is that you are going to slowly back your way into fasting. The protocol I am giving you below might need to be done over a six-month time period, easing your body into a fat-burning state. Remember, for you we want surges of hormetic stress, but not too much stress. This is why I have to step you out of some of the food and fasting styles I mentioned in prior chapters, so pay close attention to the special adaptations you need to make.

Fasting protocol for adrenal fatigue

Days 1–10: 10 hours intermittent fasting (pre-reset)
Days 11–15: no fasting (hormone feasting)
Days 16–19: 13 hours intermittent fasting (pre-reset)
Days 20–28: no fasting (hormone feasting foods)

IMMUNE SYSTEM

If you are needing a serious immune system reset, then you are going to want to lean in to a three-day water fast. This is the best fast for an overhaul of your immune system. I can't emphasize enough that if you do choose to go on a three-day water fast, then you want to take two precautions. The first is be sure you have a blood sugar and ketone reader. You need to know your numbers to make sure you are staying within safe guidelines. The second is to do your three-day water fast during one of your power phases. If you are questioning if you have low progesterone, then I would choose the first power phase window in order to not risk lowering progesterone any further.

The other fast I like for our immune systems is autophagy fasting. This fast helps to make your cells more efficient. One key element of that efficiency is that they can kill pathogens within the cell, including viruses, bacteria, and fungi. If you are catching colds more often than usual, worried about pandemic viruses, or just want to prevent the common cold, then be sure to put more autophagy fasting into your monthly cycle.

Fasting protocol for immune system reset

Days 1–5: 17 hours autophagy fasting (ketobiotic)
Days 6–9: 72 hours three-day water fast
Day 10: break water fast with four-step process
Days 11–15: 17 hours autophagy fasting (ketobiotic)
Days 16–18: 24 hours gut-reset fast (ketobiotic)
Day 19–bleed: 15 hours intermittent fasting (hormone feasting)

Endnotes

Introduction

1.   Frederick K. Ho et al., "Changes over 15 Years in the Contribution of Adiposity and Smoking to Deaths in England and Scotland," *BMC Public Health* 21, no. 1 (February 11, 2021), https://doi.org/10.1186/s12889-021-10167-3.
2.   *Lancet Diabetes & Endocrinology*, "Metabolic Health: A Priority for the Post-pandemic Era," *Lancet Diabetes & Endocrinology* 9, no. 4 (April 1, 2021): 189, https://doi.org/10.1016/s2213-8587(21)00058-9.

Chapter 1: It's Not Your Fault

1.   National Center for Health Statistics. Health, United States, 2019: Table 26. Hyattsville, MD (2021). www.cdc.gov/nchs/data/hus/2019/026-508.pdf.

Chapter 2: The Healing Power of Fasting

1. Barry Joffe and Paul Zimmet, "The Thrifty Genotype in Type 2 Diabetes: An Unfinished Symphony Moving to Its Finale?" *Endocrine* 9, no. 2 (October 1998): 139–141, https://doi.org/10.1385/endo:9:2:139.

2. Philip C. Grammaticos and Aristidis Diamantis, "Useful Known and Unknown Views of the Father of Modern Medicine, Hippocrates and His Teacher Democritus," *Hellenic Journal of Nuclear Medicine* 11, no. 1 (January–April 2008): 2–4, https://pubmed.ncbi.nlm.nih.gov/18392218/.

3. Rafael de Cabo and Mark P. Mattson, "Effects of Intermittent Fasting on Health, Aging, and Disease," *New England Journal of Medicine* 381, no. 26 (December 26, 2019): 2541–2551, https://doi.org/10.1056/nejmra1905136.

4. University of Illinois at Chicago, "Daily Fasting Works for Weight Loss, Finds Report on 16:8 Diet," ScienceDaily (June 18, 2018), www.sciencedaily.com/releases/2018/06/180618113038.htm.

5. Michael J. Wilkinson et al., "Ten-Hour Time-Restricted Eating Reduces Weight, Blood Pressure, and Atherogenic Lipids in Patients with Metabolic Syndrome," *Cell Metabolism* 31, no. 1 (January 7, 2020): 92–104, https://doi.org/10.1016/j.cmet.2019.11.004.

6. Douglas R. Green, Lorenzo Galluzzi, and Guido Kroemer, "Mitochondria and the Autophagy–Inflammation–Cell Death Axis in Organismal Aging," *Science* 333, no. 6046 (August 26, 2011): 1109–1112, https://doi.org/10.1126/science.1201940.

7. Chaysavanh Manichanh et al., "Reshaping the Gut Microbiome with Bacterial Transplantation and Antibiotic Intake," *Genome Research* 20, no. 10 (October 2010): 1411–1419, https://doi.org/10.1101/gr.107987.110.

8. Heidi Dutton et al., "Antibiotic Exposure and Risk of Weight Gain and Obesity: Protocol for a Systematic Review,"

Systematic Reviews 6, no. 169 (2017), https://doi.org/10.11 86/s13643-017-0565-9.

9. Peter J. Turnbaugh et al., "A Core Gut Microbiome in Obese and Lean Twins," *Nature* 457, no. 7228 (January 22, 2009): 480–484, https://doi.org/10.1038/nature07540.

10. Serguëi O. Fetissov, "Role of the Gut Microbiota in Host Appetite Control: Bacterial Growth to Animal Feeding Behaviour," *Nature Reviews Endocrinology* 13, no. 1 (January 2017): 11–25, https://doi.org/10.1038/nrendo.2016.150.

11. Guolin Li et al., "Intermittent Fasting Promotes White Adipose Browning and Decreases Obesity by Shaping the Gut Microbiota," *Cell Metabolism* 26, no. 4 (October 3, 2017): 672–685, https://doi.org/10.1016/j.cmet.2017.08.019.

12. Pooneh Angoorani et al., "Gut Microbiota Modulation as a Possible Mediating Mechanism for Fasting-Induced Alleviation of Metabolic Complications: A Systematic Review," *Nutrition & Metabolism* 18, no. 105 (2021), https://doi.org/10.1186/s12 986-021-00635-3.

13. Anne Trafton, "Biologists Find a Way to Boost Intestinal Stem Cell Populations," MIT News, Massachusetts Institute of Technology (March 28, 2019), https://news.mit.edu/2019/rev erse-aging-intestinal-stem-cell-0328.

14. Mehrdad Alirezaei et al., "Short-Term Fasting Induces Profound Neuronal Autophagy," *Autophagy* 6, no. 6 (August 16, 2010): 702–710, https://doi.org/10.4161/auto.6.6.12376.

15. Trafton, "Biologists Find a Way to Boost Intestinal Stem Cell Populations."

16. Cell Press, "Clinical Trial Shows Alternate-Day Fasting a Safe Alternative to Caloric Restriction," ScienceDaily (August 27, 2019), www.sciencedaily.com/releases/2019/08/1908271110 51.htm.

17. DOE/Brookhaven National Laboratory, "Food Restriction Increases Dopamine Receptors—Linked to Pleasure—in Rats,"

ScienceDaily (October 29, 2007), www.sciencedaily.com/rele
ases/2007/10/071025091036.htm.

18. Suzanne Wu, "Fasting Triggers Stem Cell Regeneration of Damaged, Old Immune System," USC News (Chia Wei-Cheng et. al, "Prolonged Fasting Reduces IGF-1/PKA to Promote Hematopoietic-Stem-Cell-Based Regeneration and Reverse Immunosuppression," *Cell Stem Cell* 14, no. 6 [June 5, 2014]), https://news.usc.edu/63669/fasting-triggers-stem-ce ll-regeneration-of-damaged-old-immune-system.

Chapter 3: Metabolic Switching: The Missing Key to Weight Loss

1.   Thomas N. Seyfried, "Cancer as a Mitochondrial Metabolic Disease," *Frontiers in Cell and Developmental Biology* 3 (July 7, 2015): 43, https://doi.org/10.3389/fcell.2015.00043.

2.   Katsuyasu Kouda and Masayuki Iki, "Beneficial Effects of Mild Stress (Hormetic Effects): Dietary Restriction and Health," *Journal of Physiological Anthropology* 29, no. 4 (2010): 127–132, https://doi.org/10.2114/jpa2.29.127.

3.   Samar H.K. Tareen et al., "Stratifying Cellular Metabolism during Weight Loss: An Interplay of Metabolism, Metabolic Flexibility and Inflammation," *Scientific Reports* 10, no. 1651 (2020), https://doi.org/10.1038/s41598-020-58358-z.

Chapter 4: Fasting a Woman's Way

1.   Bronwyn M. Graham and Mohammed R. Milad, "Blockade of Estrogen by Hormonal Contraceptives Impairs Fear Extinction in Female Rats and Women," *Biological Psychiatry* 73, no. 4 (February 15, 2013): 371–378, https://doi.org/10.1016/j.bio psych.2012.09.018.

Chapter 5: Build a Fasting Lifestyle Unique to You

1.   Sheldon Greenfield, Sherrie H. Kaplan, and John E. Ware, "Expanding Patient Involvement in Care," *Annals of Internal Medicine* 102, no. 4 (April 1985): 520–528, https://doi.org/1 0.7326/0003-4819-102-4-520.

2.   C. Jane Nikles, Alexandra M. Clavarino, and Chris B. Del Mar, "Using *N*-of-1 Trials as a Clinical Tool to Improve Prescribing," *British Journal of General Practice* 55, no. 512 (March 2005): 175–180, https://bjgp.org/content/55/512/175.

Chapter 6: Foods That Support Your Hormones

1. Cameron Faustman et al., "Ten Years Post-GAO Assessment, FDA Remains Uninformed of Potentially Harmful GRAS Substances in Foods," *Critical Reviews in Food Science and Nutrition* 61, no. 8 (2021): 1260–1268, https://doi.org/10.1080/10408398.2020.1756217.

2. David Andrews, "Synthetic Ingredients in Natural Flavors and Natural Flavors in Artificial Flavors," EWG (Environmental Working Group), www.ewg.org/foodscores/content/natural-vs-artificial-flavors.

3. Kamal Niaz, Elizabeta Zaplatic, and Jonathan Spoor, "Extensive Use of Monosodium Glutamate: A Threat to Public Health?" *EXCLI Journal* 17 (March 19, 2018): 273–278, https://doi.org/10.17179/excli2018-1092.

4. "Acrylamide and Cancer Risk," National Cancer Institute, accessed April 26, 2022, www.cancer.gov/about-cancer/causes-prevention/risk/diet/acrylamide-fact-sheet.

5. National Institutes of Health, "Women's Cholesterol Levels Vary with Phase of Menstrual Cycle" (August 10, 2010), www.nih.gov/news-events/news-releases/womens-cholesterol-levels-vary-phase-menstrual-cycle.

6. Sarah J. Nechuta et al., "Soy Food Intake after Diagnosis of Breast Cancer and Survival: An In-Depth Analysis of Combined Evidence from Cohort Studies of US and Chinese Women," *American Journal of Clinical Nutrition* 96, no. 1 (July 2012): 123–132, https://doi.org/10.3945/ajcn.112.035972.

7. Elena Volpi et al., "Is the Optimal Level of Protein Intake for Older Adults Greater than the Recommended Dietary Allowance?" *Journals of Gerontology Series A: Biological Sciences and Medical Sciences* 68, no. 6 (June 2013): 677–681, https://doi.org/10.1093/gerona/gls229.

8. Seo-Jin Yang et al., "Antioxidant and Immune-Enhancing Effects of Probiotic *Lactobacillus plantarum* 200655 Isolated from Kimchi," *Food Science and Biotechnology* 28, no. 2

(April 2019): 491–499, https://doi.org/10.1007/s10068-018-0473-3.

9. María García-Burgos et al., "New Perspectives in Fermented Dairy Products and Their Health Relevance," *Journal of Functional Foods* 72 (September 2020): 104059, https://doi.org/10.1016/j.jff.2020.104059.

10. Elizabeth I. Opara and Magali Chohan, "Culinary Herbs and Spices: Their Bioactive Properties, the Contribution of Polyphenols and the Challenges in Deducing Their True Health Benefits," *International Journal of Molecular Sciences* 15, no. 10 (October 22, 2014): 19183–19202, https://doi.org/10.3390/ijms151019183.

11. Shakir Ali et al., "Eugenol-Rich Fraction of *Syzygium aromaticum* (Clove) Reverses Biochemical and Histopathological Changes in Liver Cirrhosis and Inhibits Hepatic Cell Proliferation," *Journal of Cancer Prevention* 19, no. 4 (December 2014): 288–300, https://doi.org/10.15430/jcp.2014.19.4.288.

12. Joe Alcock, Carlo C. Maley, and C. Athena Aktipis, "Is Eating Behavior Manipulated by the Gastrointestinal Microbiota? Evolutionary Pressures and Potential Mechanisms," *BioEssays* 36, no. 10 (October 2014): 940–949, https://doi.org/10.1002/bies.201400071.

Chapter 9: How to Break a Fast

1. Brad Jon Schoenfeld and Alan Albert Aragon, "How Much Protein Can the Body Use in a Single Meal for Muscle-Building? Implications for Daily Protein Distribution," *Journal of the International Society of Sports Nutrition* 15 (February 27, 2018): 10, https://doi.org/10.1186/s12970-018-0215-1.

2. Tibor I. Krisko et al., "Dissociation of Adaptive Thermogenesis from Glucose Homeostasis in Microbiome-Deficient Mice," *Cell Metabolism* 31, no. 3 (March 3, 2020): 592–604, https://doi.org/10.1016/j.cmet.2020.01.012.

3. Pamela M. Peeke et al., "Effect of Time Restricted Eating on Body Weight and Fasting Glucose in Participants with Obesity: Results of a Randomized, Controlled, Virtual Clinical Trial," *Nutrition & Diabetes* 11, no. 1 (January 15, 2021): 6, https://doi.org/10.1038/s41387-021-00149-0.

Chapter 10: Hacks That Make Fasting Effortless

1. Fereidoun Azizi, "Effect of Dietary Composition on Fasting-Induced Changes in Serum Thyroid Hormones and Thyrotropin," *Metabolism* 27, no. 8 (August 1, 1978): 935–942, https://doi.org/10.1016/0026-0495(78)90137-3.

Bibliography

Alcock, Joe, Carlo C. Maley, and C. Athena Aktipis. "Is Eating Behavior Manipulated by the Gastrointestinal Microbiota? Evolutionary Pressures and Potential Mechanisms." *BioEssays* 36, no. 10 (October 2014): 940–49. https://doi.org/10.1002/bies.201400071.

Ali, Shakir, Ram Prasad, Amena Mahmood, Indusmita Routray, Tijjani Salihu Shinkafi, Kazim Sahin, and Omer Kucuk. "Eugenol-Rich Fraction of *Syzygium aromaticum* (Clove) Reverses Biochemical and Histopathological Changes in Liver Cirrhosis and Inhibits Hepatic Cell Proliferation." *Journal of Cancer Prevention* 19, no. 4 (December 2014): 288–300. https://doi.org/10.15430/jcp.2014.19.4.288.

Alirezaei, Mehrdad, Christopher C. Kemball, Claudia T. Flynn, Malcolm R. Wood, J. Lindsay Whitton, and William B. Kiosses. "Short-Term Fasting Induces Profound Neuronal Autophagy." *Autophagy* 6, no. 6 (August 16, 2010): 702–10. https://doi.org/10.4161/auto.6.6.12376.

Andrews, David. "Synthetic Ingredients in Natural Flavors and Natural Flavors in Artificial Flavors." EWG. Environmental Working Group. Accessed April 26, 2022. https://www.ewg.org/foodscores/content/natural-vs-artificial-flavors/.

Angoorani, Pooneh, Hanieh-Sadat Ejtahed, Shirin Hasani-Ranjbar, Seyed Davar Siadat, Ahmad Reza Soroush, and Bagher Larijani. "Gut Microbiota Modulation as a Possible Mediating Mechanism for Fasting-Induced Alleviation of Metabolic Complications: A Systematic Review." *Nutrition & Metabolism*

18, no. 105 (2021). https://doi.org/10.1186/s12986-021-00635-3.

Azizi, Fereidoun. "Effect of Dietary Composition on Fasting-Induced Changes in Serum Thyroid Hormones and Thyrotropin." *Metabolism* 27, no. 8 (August 1, 1978): 935–42. https://doi.org/10.1016/0026-0495(78)90137-3.

Cell Press. "Clinical Trial Shows Alternate-Day Fasting a Safe Alternative to Caloric Restriction." ScienceDaily (August 27, 2019). https://www.sciencedaily.com/releases/2019/08/190827111051.htm.

de Cabo, Rafael, and Mark P. Mattson. "Effects of Intermittent Fasting on Health, Aging, and Disease." *New England Journal of Medicine* 381, no. 26 (December 26, 2019): 2541–51. https://doi.org/10.1056/nejmra1905136.

DOE/Brookhaven National Laboratory. "Food Restriction Increases Dopamine Receptors—Linked to Pleasure—in Rats." ScienceDaily (October 29, 2007). https://www.sciencedaily.com/releases/2007/10/071025091036.htm.

Dutton, Heidi, Mary-Anne Doyle, C. Arianne Buchan, Shuhiba Mohammad, Kristi B. Adamo, Risa Shorr, and Dean A. Fergusson. "Antibiotic Exposure and Risk of Weight Gain and Obesity: Protocol for a Systematic Review." *Systematic Reviews* 6, no. 169 (2017). https://doi.org/10.1186/s13643-017-0565-9.

Faustman, Cameron, Daniel Aaron, Nicole Negowetti, and Emily Broad Leib. "Ten Years Post-GAO Assessment, FDA Remains Uninformed of Potentially Harmful GRAS Substances in Foods." *Critical Reviews in Food Science and Nutrition* 61, no. 8 (2021): 1260–68. https://doi.org/10.1080/10408398.2020.1756217.

Fetissov, Serguei O. "Role of the Gut Microbiota in Host Appetite Control: Bacterial Growth to Animal Feeding Behaviour." *Nature Reviews Endocrinology* 13, no. 1 (January 2017): 11–25. https://doi.org/10.1038/nrendo.2016.150.

García-Burgos, María, Jorge Moreno-Fernández, María J.M. Alférez, Javier Díaz-Castro, and Inmaculada López-Aliaga. "New Perspectives in Fermented Dairy Products and Their Health Relevance." *Journal of Functional Foods* 72 (September 2020): 104059. https://doi.org/10.1016/j.jff.2020.104059.

Graham, Bronwyn M., and Mohammed R. Milad. "Blockade of Estrogen by Hormonal Contraceptives Impairs Fear Extinction in Female Rats and Women." *Biological Psychiatry* 73, no. 4 (February 15, 2013): 371–78. https://doi.org/10.1016/j.biopsych.2012.09.018.

Grammaticos, Philip C., and Aristidis Diamantis. "Useful Known and Unknown Views of the Father of Modern Medicine, Hippocrates and His Teacher Democritus." *Hellenic Journal of Nuclear Medicine* 11, no. 1 (January–April 2008): 2–4. https://pubmed.ncbi.nlm.nih.gov/18392218/.

Green, Douglas R., Lorenzo Galluzzi, and Guido Kroemer. "Mitochondria and the Autophagy–Inflammation–Cell Death Axis in Organismal Aging." *Science* 333, no. 6046 (August 26, 2011): 1109–12. https://doi.org/10.1126/science.1201940.

Greenfield, Sheldon, Sherrie H. Kaplan, and John E. Ware. "Expanding Patient Involvement in Care." *Annals of Internal Medicine* 102, no. 4 (April 1, 1985): 520–28. https://doi.org/10.7326/0003-4819-102-4-520.

Ho, Frederick K., Carlos Celis-Morales, Fanny Petermann-Rocha, Solange Liliana Parra-Soto, James Lewsey, Daniel Mackay, and Jill P. Pell. "Changes over 15 Years in the Contribution of

Adiposity and Smoking to Deaths in England and Scotland." *BMC Public Health* 21, no. 1 (February 11, 2021). https://doi.org/10.1186/s12889-021-10167-3.

Joffe, Barry, and Paul Zimmet. "The Thrifty Genotype in Type 2 Diabetes: An Unfinished Symphony Moving to Its Finale?" *Endocrine* 9, no. 2 (October 1998): 139–41. https://doi.org/10.1385/endo:9:2:139.

Kouda, Katsuyasu, and Masayuki Iki. "Beneficial Effects of Mild Stress (Hormetic Effects): Dietary Restriction and Health." *Journal of Physiological Anthropology* 29, no. 4 (2010): 127–32. https://doi.org/10.2114/jpa2.29.127.

Krisko, Tibor I., Hayley T. Nicholls, Curtis J. Bare, Corey D. Holman, Gregory G. Putzel, Robert S. Jansen, Natalie Sun, Kyu Y. Rhee, Alexander S. Banks, and David E. Cohen. "Dissociation of Adaptive Thermogenesis from Glucose Homeostasis in Microbiome-Deficient Mice." *Cell Metabolism* 31, no. 3 (March 3, 2020): 592–604. https://doi.org/10.1016/j.cmet.2020.01.012.

Lancet Diabetes & Endocrinology. "Metabolic Health: A Priority for the Post-pandemic Era." *Lancet Diabetes & Endocrinology* 9, no. 4 (April 1, 2021): 189. https://doi.org/10.1016/s2213-8587(21)00058-9.

Li, Guolin, Cen Xie, Siyu Lu, Robert G. Nichols, Yuan Tian, Licen Li, Daxeshkumar Patel, et al. "Intermittent Fasting Promotes White Adipose Browning and Decreases Obesity by Shaping the Gut Microbiota." *Cell Metabolism* 26, no. 4 (October 3, 2017): 672–85. https://doi.org/10.1016/j.cmet.2017.08.019.

Manichanh, Chaysavanh, Jens Reeder, Prudence Gibert, Encarna Varela, Marta Llopis, Maria Antolin, Roderic Guigo, Rob Knight, and Francisco Guarner. "Reshaping the Gut Microbiome with Bacterial Transplantation and Antibiotic Intake." *Genome*

Research 20, no. 10 (October 2010): 1411–19. https://doi.org/1 0.1101/gr.107987.110.

National Cancer Institute. "Acrylamide and Cancer Risk." National Cancer Institute. Accessed April 26, 2022. https://ww w.cancer.gov/about-cancer/causes-prevention/risk/diet/acrylami de-fact-sheet.

National Institutes of Health. "Women's Cholesterol Levels Vary with Phase of Menstrual Cycle." U.S. Department of Health and Human Services (August 10, 2010). https://www.nih.gov/news-events/news-releases/womens-cholesterol-levels-vary-phase-m enstrual-cycle.

Nechuta, Sarah J., Bette J. Caan, Wendy Y. Chen, Wei Lu, Zhi Chen, Marilyn L. Kwan, Shirley W. Flatt, et al. "Soy Food Intake after Diagnosis of Breast Cancer and Survival: An In-Depth Analysis of Combined Evidence from Cohort Studies of US and Chinese Women." *American Journal of Clinical Nutrition* 96, no. 1 (July 2012): 123–32. https://doi.org/10.3945/ajcn.112.035972.

Niaz, Kamal, Elizabeta Zaplatic, and Jonathan Spoor. "Extensive Use of Monosodium Glutamate: A Threat to Public Health?" *EXCLI Journal* 17 (March 19, 2018): 273–78. https://doi.org/10. 17179/excli2018-1092.

Nikles, C. Jane, Alexandra M. Clavarino, and Chris B. Del Mar. "Using *N*-of-1 Trials as a Clinical Tool to Improve Prescribing." *British Journal of General Practice* 55, no. 512 (March 2005): 175–80. https://bjgp.org/content/55/512/175.

Opara, Elizabeth I., and Magali Chohan. "Culinary Herbs and Spices: Their Bioactive Properties, the Contribution of Polyphenols and the Challenges in Deducing Their True Health Benefits." *International Journal of Molecular Sciences* 15, no. 10

(October 22, 2014): 19183–202. https://doi.org/10.3390/ijms151019183.

Peeke, Pamela M., Frank L. Greenway, Sonja K. Billes, Dachuan Zhang, and Ken Fujioka. "Effect of Time Restricted Eating on Body Weight and Fasting Glucose in Participants with Obesity: Results of a Randomized, Controlled, Virtual Clinical Trial." *Nutrition & Diabetes* 11, no. 1 (January 15, 2021): 6. https://doi.org/10.1038/s41387-021-00149-0.

Schoenfeld, Brad Jon, and Alan Albert Aragon. "How Much Protein Can the Body Use in a Single Meal for Muscle-Building? Implications for Daily Protein Distribution." *Journal of the International Society of Sports Nutrition* 15, no. 1 (2018): 10. https://doi.org/10.1186/s12970-018-0215-1.

Seyfried, Thomas N. "Cancer as a Mitochondrial Metabolic Disease." *Frontiers in Cell and Developmental Biology* 3 (July 7, 2015): 43. https://doi.org/10.3389/fcell.2015.00043.

Tareen, Samar H.K., Martina Kutmon, Theo M. de Kok, Edwin C. Mariman, Marleen A. van Baak, Chris T. Evelo, Michiel E. Adriaens, and Ilja C. W. Arts. "Stratifying Cellular Metabolism during Weight Loss: An Interplay of Metabolism, Metabolic Flexibility and Inflammation." *Scientific Reports* 10, no. 1651 (2020). https://doi.org/10.1038/s41598-020-58358-z.

Trafton, Anne. "Biologists Find a Way to Boost Intestinal Stem Cell Populations." MIT News, Massachusetts Institute of Technology (March 28, 2019). https://news.mit.edu/2019/reverse-aging-intestinal-stem-cell-0328.

Turnbaugh, Peter J., Micah Hamady, Tanya Yatsunenko, Brandi L. Cantarel, Alexis Duncan, Ruth E. Ley, Mitchell L. Sogin, et al. "A Core Gut Microbiome in Obese and Lean Twins." *Nature* 457, no.

7228 (January 22, 2009): 480–84. https://doi.org/10.1038/natu
re07540.

University of Illinois at Chicago. "Daily Fasting Works for Weight Loss, Finds Report on 16:8 Diet." ScienceDaily (June 18, 2018). https://www.sciencedaily.com/releases/2018/06/18061811303 8.htm.

Volpi, Elena, Wayne W. Campbell, Johanna T. Dwyer, Mary Ann Johnson, Gordon L. Jensen, John E. Morley, and Robert R. Wolfe. "Is the Optimal Level of Protein Intake for Older Adults Greater than the Recommended Dietary Allowance?" *Journals of Gerontology Series A: Biological Sciences and Medical Sciences* 68, no. 6 (June 2013): 677–81. https://doi.org/10.1093/geron a/gls229.

Wilkinson, Michael J., Emily N. C. Manoogian, Adena Zadourian, Hannah Lo, Savannah Fakhouri, Azarin Shoghi, Xinran Wang, et al. "Ten-Hour Time-Restricted Eating Reduces Weight, Blood Pressure, and Atherogenic Lipids in Patients with Metabolic Syndrome." *Cell Metabolism* 31, no. 1 (January 7, 2020): 92–104. https://doi.org/10.1016/j.cmet.2019.11.004.

Wu, Suzanne. "Fasting Triggers Stem Cell Regeneration of Damaged, Old Immune System." USC News. *Cell Stem Cell* 14, no. 6 (June 5, 2014). https://news.usc.edu/63669/fasting-trigge rs-stem-cell-regeneration-of-damaged-old-immune-system/.

Yang, Seo-Jin, Ji-Eun Lee, Sung-Min Lim, Yu-Jin Kim, Na-Kyoung Lee, and HyunDong Paik. "Antioxidant and Immune-Enhancing Effects of Probiotic *Lactobacillus plantarum* 200655 Isolated from Kimchi." *Food Science and Biotechnology* 28, no. 2 (April 2019): 491–99. https://doi.org/10.1007/s10068-018-0473-3.

Recipe Index

Note: Recipe titles followed by (V) indicate vegetarian selections. Page numbers in parentheses indicate intermittent references.

C

D

E

K

L

M

T

W

Z

General Index

A

G

Acknowledgments

Writing a book is not a solo journey. An idea sparks in an author's mind that has stemmed from thousands of conversations, a meritage of life experiences, hours of rabbit holes of research, and a deep desire to shed light on the challenges that face the world today.

As I sit here thinking deeply about the people to acknowledge who have contributed to this book, I realize that this book is truly a collaboration of people, ideas, and dreams that united to bring you the words that live on these pages.

First, I must acknowledge all the powerful women whose energy has influenced my thoughts about hormones and fasting. When I started to teach the world the wonders of fasting, we didn't have a lot of fasting answers for women. So many of you poured onto my social media platforms searching for those answers. To the millions of women who have watched my videos, asked questions, left comments, and told me the fasting hurdles you were encountering, I say thank you. Too many of you are feeling lost and at the end of your health rope. I deeply appreciate that every video I asked you to comment on, question, or to share your struggles, you did. You opened your hearts, expressed your frustrations, and acknowledged your desperate pleas to find a new health path that was unique to you. When I asked you to be there for the community, share your fasting wins, inspire new fasters, or offer words of encouragement, you showed up. My team and I have read every message, responded to each one of your comments, and heard every cry you have left on my socials. Please know, from the bottom of my heart, I am cheering you on. This book is for you.

When the pandemic hit, I was blessed to be in an author mastermind group with Marianne Williamson. We met biweekly on Zoom, often for hours, as she poured her wisdom into us. Marianne, you changed the way I viewed the responsibility of an author. You are truly a master of this craft, and I feel so blessed to have had a unique glimpse into your writing wizardry.

This book truly became a reality the day I met my literary agent, Stephanie Tade. Stephanie, I had a mission in my heart and you saw it. Thank you for seeing my vision so clearly. I appreciate your patience, wisdom, and guidance through this process. Kathy Huck, editor extraordinaire, I am forever grateful for you. Not only did your wisdom make me a better writer, but your knack for taking my ridiculously enthusiastic thoughts and smoothing them into silky sentences was greatly appreciated. To the Hay House team, especially Melody Guy, thank you for seeing what women needed in a fasting book. I feel so supported and blessed to be part of the Hay House family. What an honor to be on this journey with you.

Walking the path of health with another is a very intimate experience. There is a lot of trust, openness, and vulnerability required. To the women I have personally coached over the years, thank you for inviting me into your worlds. I know healing can often feel like a turbulent ride that has no clear path. Thank you for trusting me. It has been my deepest honor to witness you getting your lives back.

As I was researching and writing this book, several other amazing humans entered my world. Jesse, I didn't think I could feel more excited about fasting, until I met you. Thank you for sparking the International Fasting Day idea, your relentless support of my fasting mission, your enthusiasm for the empowerment of women, and for modeling what the life of a happy human looks like. Kat, I so appreciate you seeing my heart for serving humanity so early in our connection. Your infectious spirit and commitment to the millions that follow you spoke so deeply to me. I love uniting our missions. LeAnn, I have never seen a human more dedicated to her health journey than you. Your willingness to do "all the things" has motivated me to dig deeper, looking for solutions for not only you but all women. What an honor it's been to walk alongside you in your healing journey. You have deeply touched my soul, stretched me to keep researching, and taught me the power of wearing your heart on your sleeve.

To my amazing team who are boots on the ground doing the work needed to serve the needs of our community. From the bottom of my heart, thank you. I am incredibly honored to be serving health to the world with you all. Jessica, Lynda, Debbie, Rachel, Paige, Eliza, Myta, Christiane, Andrea, Denise, Dana, Marisol, and Isaac, thank you for putting in the work needed to make my crazy desire to change health care for women into a reality.

A massive thank you to all the amazing colleagues and mentors who have shaped the way I view the human body and its vast ability to self-heal. I am eternally grateful to you for all the baby neurons you grew in my brain by sharing your perspectives, research, and philosophies with me. A special shout-out to Dr. Carrie Jones, who graciously brainstormed the Fasting Cycle with me when it was in its early stages.

Lastly, to my family. You are my everything. Seriously, life makes sense when I am with you. Bodhi and Pax, the depth in which you show up in life moves me more than words could ever appropriately express. My greatest honor has been being your mom. My sweet hubby, Sequoia, who listens to me more than any other human on the planet. I could not have written this book without you. Thank you for being my muse.

About the Author

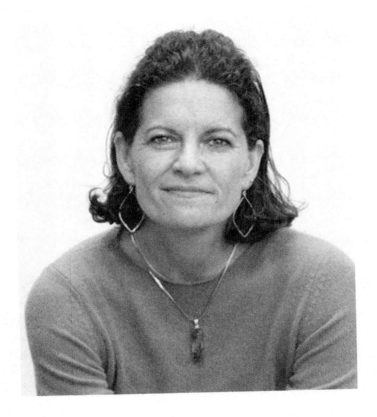

Dr. Mindy H. Pelz, DC, is a best-selling author, keynote speaker, and nutrition and functional health expert who has spent over two decades helping thousands of people successfully reclaim their health. She is a recognized leader in the alternative health field and a pioneer in the fasting movement, teaching the principles of a fasting lifestyle, diet variation, detox, hormones, and more. Her popular YouTube channel, where she regularly updates followers on the latest science-backed tools and techniques to help them reset their health, has had more than 24 million lifetime views. She is the host of one of the leading science podcasts, *The Resetter Podcast*, and the author of three best-selling books, *The Menopause Reset*, *The Reset Factor*, and *The Reset Factor Kitchen*. Dr. Mindy has appeared on national shows like *Extra TV* and *The Doctors*, and has been featured in *Muscle & Fitness*, *Well + Good*, *SheKnows*, *Healthline*, and more.

To learn more about Dr. Mindy and her work, visit drmindypelz.com.

Printed in Great Britain
by Amazon

20438153R00217